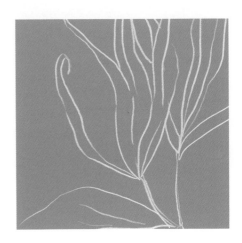

aromatherapy
a beginner's guide

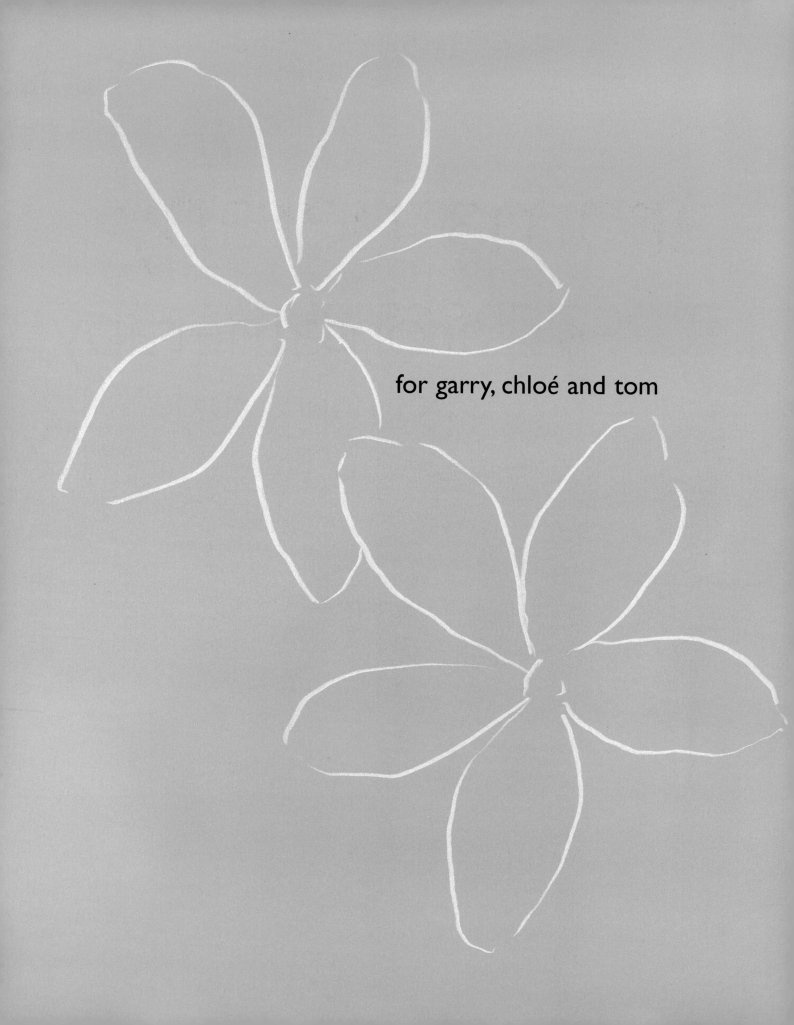

for garry, chloé and tom

aromatherapy
a beginner's guide

Denise Whichello Brown

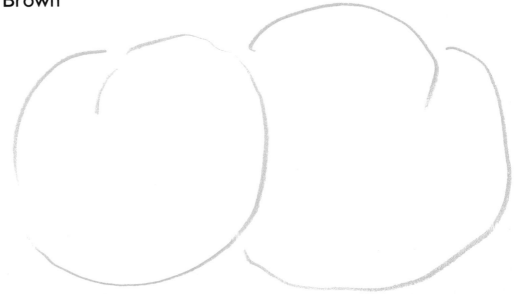

Published by SILVERDALE BOOKS
An imprint of Bookmart Ltd
Registered number 2372865
Trading as Bookmart Ltd
Desford Road
Enderby
Leicester LE19 4AD

© 2003 D&S Books Ltd

D&S Books Ltd
Kerswell,
Parkham Ash, Bideford
Devon, England
EX39 5PR

e-mail us at:-
enquiries@dsbooks.fsnet.co.uk

This edition printed 2003

ISBN 1-856057-41-0

Book Code DS0069 Aromatherapy

Creative Director: Sarah King
Editor: Anna Southgate
Project editor: Judith Millidge
Photographer: Colin Bowling
Designer: Axis Design Editions

Printed in China

1 3 5 7 9 10 8 6 4 2

contents

introduction

introduction to aromatherapy

The natural healing art of aromatherapy is an excellent way to promote optimum health and vitality. Aromatherapy uses pure essential oils to balance the body's equilibrium and to improve mental and physical health. Many common ailments may be treated and prevented simply, safely and successfully. Everyday problems such as sore throats, coughs and colds, headaches, difficulty in relaxing and sleeping, musculo-skeletal complaints, digestive problems such as indigestion and constipation, skin disorders and many other problems all respond remarkably well to aromatherapy. This book will provide you with the necessary tools to alleviate everyday health challenges that may present themselves. You will be able to practise the art of aromatherapy in your home safely and effectively.

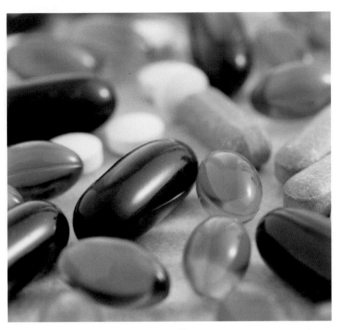

Conventional medicines may have unwanted side-effects.

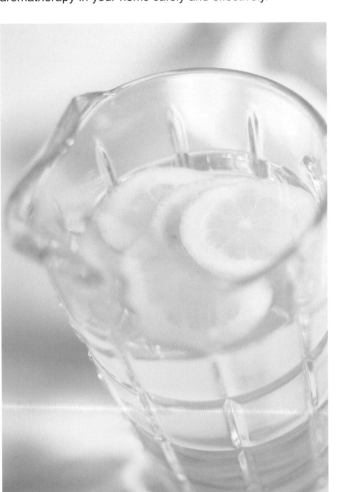

Use lemon in water for a gargle to combat a sore throat.

When used in the appropriate dilution, pure essential oils do not produce distressing side-effects in the same way as conventional medications may do. For instance, the over-use of antibiotics can result in thrush, painkillers may lead to constipation, and anti-inflammatory drugs can have an adverse effect on the stomach. I am not trying to suggest that this book should be used to diagnose and prescribe, which is, of course, the prerogative of a doctor. Any health problems that do occur should always be checked out by a medically qualified doctor, particularly if they are persistent or if the presenting symptoms are out of the ordinary. But next time you have a headache reach for the lavender and peppermint first instead of painkillers, and if you have a sore throat try a gargle with lemon. The results will surprise you and give you the confidence to use essential oils as part of your daily life.

chapter one

what are essential oils?

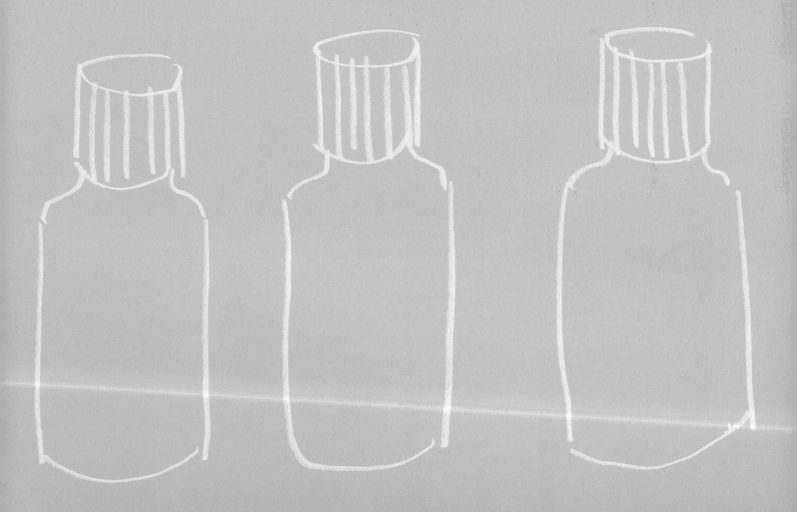

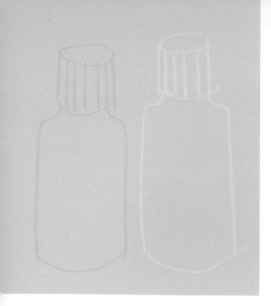

what are essential oils?

essential oils can only be produced by nature: they are the 'essence' or 'life force' of plants — some even consider them to be the 'soul'.

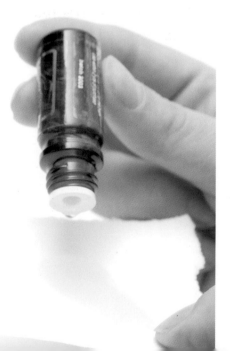

Essential oils give each plant its own unique fragrance. As you brush past a lavender or rosemary bush in your garden or whilst out walking, when you rub a lemon balm or mint leaf between your fingers, or as you smell the beautiful fragrance of a rose you are experiencing the joy of essential oils as they are released into the atmosphere.

Essential oils are also volatile. The word 'volatile' is derived from the Latin *volare* meaning to fly. In relation to essential oils, volatile refers to the fact that they evaporate (i.e. turn from a liquid to a gas) at room temperature or higher. This is one of the reasons that we can smell more aromas in the summer than in any other season of the year, as the hot weather releases the fragrance of the essential oils. In the winter when it is cooler, the essential oils are less likely to evaporate, so we do not pick up their precious scents so easily. No wonder that we all feel so much better in the summer than in the winter!

Essential oils are not only natural, highly fragrant and volatile, they are also non-oily, despite their name. A good test of the purity of these aromatic substances is that they do not leave a greasy mark on a piece of paper. Due to the high price of certain essential oils, some suppliers adulterate them by mixing them with a vegetable oil. So if it feels oily or leaves a greasy mark on paper it is not a pure essential oil — watch out for this one! There are a few exceptions to this rule, however, such as myrrh and patchouli.

Other characteristics shared by essential oils are that they are soluble in oils, fats and pure alcohol, but they are only partially soluble in water. Essential oils are also flammable and are damaged by light, heat, air and moisture. With these factors in mind, it is worth consulting the section later in this book (page 14) on how to care for your precious essential oils.

The blotting paper test assesses the oiliness of an essential oil.

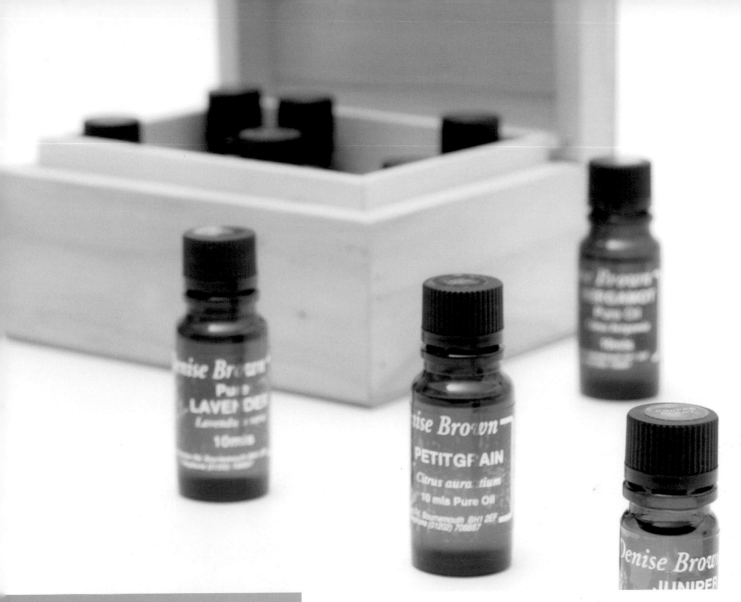

They are contained in the glandular cells, hairs, and sacs of different plants. For example:

- flowers ⟶ rose, neroli
- leaves ⟶ eucalyptus, peppermint
- wood ⟶ sandalwood
- fruits ⟶ lemon, orange
- berries ⟶ juniper
- twigs ⟶ petitgrain
- roots ⟶ ginger
- seeds ⟶ angelica
- gum ⟶ myrrh

where essential oils are found

It is interesting that more than one oil can sometimes be extracted from different parts of a particular plant, angelica seed and angelica root, for example .Neroli is derived from the blossom of the orange tree, orange from the fruit and petitgrain from the leaves and twigs.

There is an enormous difference in the amount of essential oil that is present in a plant. On average there is a yield of about 1%–2%. A 1% yield indicates that 100 kilos of plant material are required to produce 1 litre of essential oil, whereas a 2 % yield would be 2 litres of essential oil per 100 kilos. An oil such as the highly expensive rose oil yields just 0.01% essential oil. No wonder it is so costly! A cheaper oil, such as lemon or lavender, will have a higher yield. Therefore, if a supplier's oils are more or less the same price then they are unlikely to be genuine.

how are essential oils produced?

True essential oils may only be obtained by the methods of **distillation** or **expression.**

steam distillation process

Steam distillation is by far the most widely used and most economical method. The plant is heated by water or steam in a still which causes the cell structure to rupture and frees the essential oil. The steam carrying the aromatic molecules is cooled to produce a mixture of oil and water. The essential oil is then separated and bottled.

expression process

This method of extraction is employed for obtaining oil from citrus fruits such as lemon, orange, bergamot and mandarin, as their oil is present in the rind of the fruit. The expression process was originally carried out by hand, but now mechanical presses are employed.

The rind of citrus fruit is the most aromatic part of the plant.

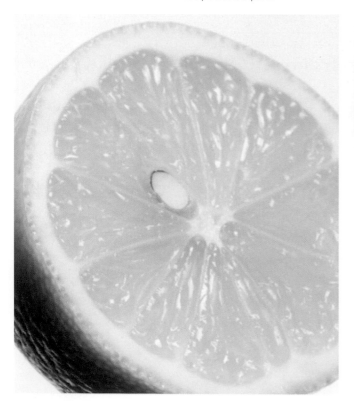

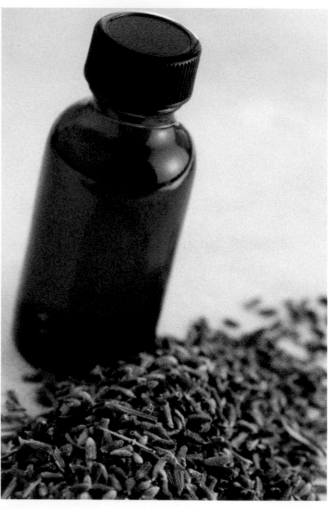

Lavender

other processes

Other processes do not yield true essential oils. They include solvent extraction, which produces absolutes, resinoids, enfleurage, carbon dioxide extraction, percolation and maceration.

Essential oils that have been extracted via the process of distillation or expression are the purest and are most commonly used for the purposes of aromatherapy. Oils obtained by solvent extraction are primarily used by the perfume and food industries.

pure or impure?

Unfortunately essential oil traders supply mainly to the perfume and the food industries which are more concerned with fragrance or flavour rather than the oils' therapeutic effects, and some essential oils may have been adulterated and are not always genuine. Naturally, for the purposes of aromatherapy the oils should be as pure and therefore as therapeutic as possible.

Synthetic oils are not suitable for aromatherapy. Always read labels carefully – words such as 'nature identical', 'fragrance' or 'perfume' indicate synthetic essential oils. Such oils may cause unpleasant side-effects such as rashes, redness or irritations. Special procedures such as gas liquid chromatography (GLC) are employed to assess the purity of essential oils.

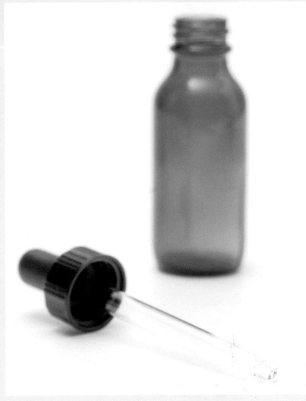

A pipette.

buying essential oils

- Do try to find an established supplier.
- Do look out for a recommendation.
- Do find an aromatherapy specialist.
- Do ask if there is a qualified aromatherapist available.
- Do check that the oils are batch-numbered in case of complaint.
- Do compare the prices of the oils. There should be a wide difference in prices. Essential oil of jasmine or rose should be far more expensive than lavender or lemon.
- Do ask if the oils are sold in glass amber-coloured bottles (to protect them from damage by sunlight).
- Do ask if the oils are 100% pure.
- Do read labels carefully – check for words such as 'nature identical' or 'fragrance' indicating impurity.

- Do check that the bottles have flow reduction inserts to enable you to accurately measure the number of drops.
- Do look for bottles without rubber stoppers or pipettes since essential oils will destroy rubber.
- Do trust your nose. The more you use the essential oils the more easily you will be able to detect a 'true' essential oil.
- Do put a few drops on a piece of blotting paper or fairly thick paper and allow it to dry. If a mark is left behind be suspicious.
- Do rub a drop of essential oil between your thumb and forefinger. There should NOT be a greasy feel.
- Do buy just a very small selection of oils to begin with. If you are happy with the quality then purchase more.

taking care of your oils

Your precious bottles of essential oils will last a long time. Bearing in mind that you will only be using a few drops at a time and that the average 10 ml (⅓ fl oz) bottle contains 200 drops, one bottle will last for ages. It is therefore important to store them properly. In the right conditions, essential oils will last on average for at least two years, and may last for as long as five years. Some essential oils are like a good wine and are considered to improve with age! Citrus oils, which are extremely cheap anyway, have a shorter shelf life, and absolutes (extracted via solvent extraction) have a tendency to thicken with age so the aroma of the solvent is more noticeable.

Once essential oils have been diluted in a blend containing a vegetable oil, the shelf life is reduced dramatically to between three and six months. Blends are always at their best when freshly prepared – this is why it's not a good idea to buy a blend from a shop as you do not know how long ago it was blended or by whom.

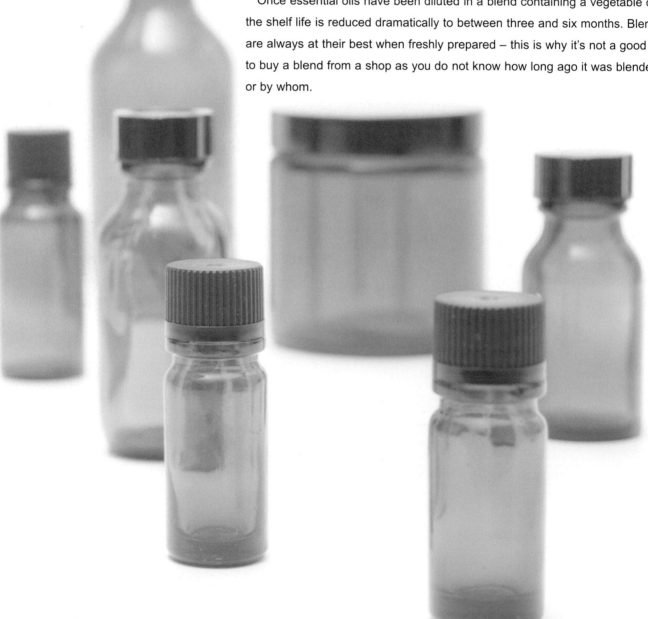

tips for storage

- Keep your oils in amber glass bottles. This is to protect them from damage by natural light.
- Do not place them in direct sunlight – e.g. on a sunny window sill.
- Do not decant them into plastic bottles, as they will buckle.
- Keep your oils at an even temperature. They are adversely affected by very hot or very cold conditions.
- Keep them out of reach of young children. Essential oils are extremely potent. If they are swallowed, seek medical advice immediately.
- Make sure that the bottles have flow reduction inserts in them to allow you to gauge the number of drops. You should not keep them in bottles with rubber stoppers or bottles with pipettes as the rubber parts will be destroyed by the essential oils.

- Always replace tops immediately after use. Remember essential oils are extremely volatile and will evaporate readily.
- Do not put them near a naked flame. Remember they are flammable.
- Never put bottles onto a polished or plastic surface, as accidental spills of essential oils will damage such surfaces.
- Store essential oils away from homeopathic medicines. Certain oils, such as tea tree, peppermint and eucalyptus may affect homeopathic remedies.

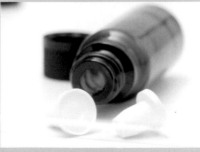

Flow inserts control the number of drops leaving the bottle.

how do essential oils work?

The primary ways that essential oils are able to enter the body are via the skin or the nose.

Our skin is designed to let some substances in and to keep others out. Essential oils, unlike many other substances, are able to penetrate through the skin because of their small molecules.

They are absorbed into the bloodstream from where they may be transported to any organs or structures where they are needed. They are then excreted in the urine, faeces or via our perspiration or our breath. If you find this difficult to believe, then rub a clove of garlic on the sole of your foot. After about 15 minutes you (or your partner!) will detect the smell of garlic on your breath.

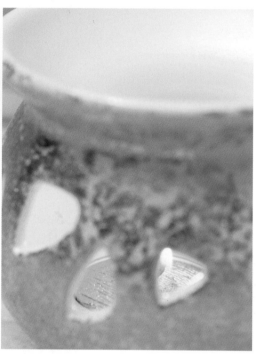

Oil burner.

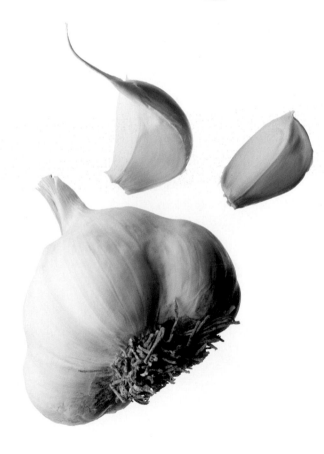

Try the garlic test!

Our nose-brain connection is very powerful. When we inhale an essential oil it affects the limbic part of our brain which is where our emotions and mood functions are seated. Aromas and memories are very strongly linked. Perhaps the smell of lavender will remind you of your favourite grandmother (or the grandmother you were not particularly fond of!). Whenever a smell, such as freshly baked bread, the aroma of cigar smoke, freshly ground coffee, a perfume that your mother wore or your father's aftershave, evokes a memory this is because of the nose-brain connection. Essential oils are potent mood-changers. For instance, chamomile can turn anger to calmness, neroli can dispel depression and black pepper can fill you with determination and courage. It is this connection that totally fascinates and amazes my students when they begin to work on clients. Many a student has uttered the words, 'I would never have believed how powerful essential oils are'. You, too, will marvel at the ancient therapeutic art of aromatherapy.

Aromas and smells can evoke powerful memories....

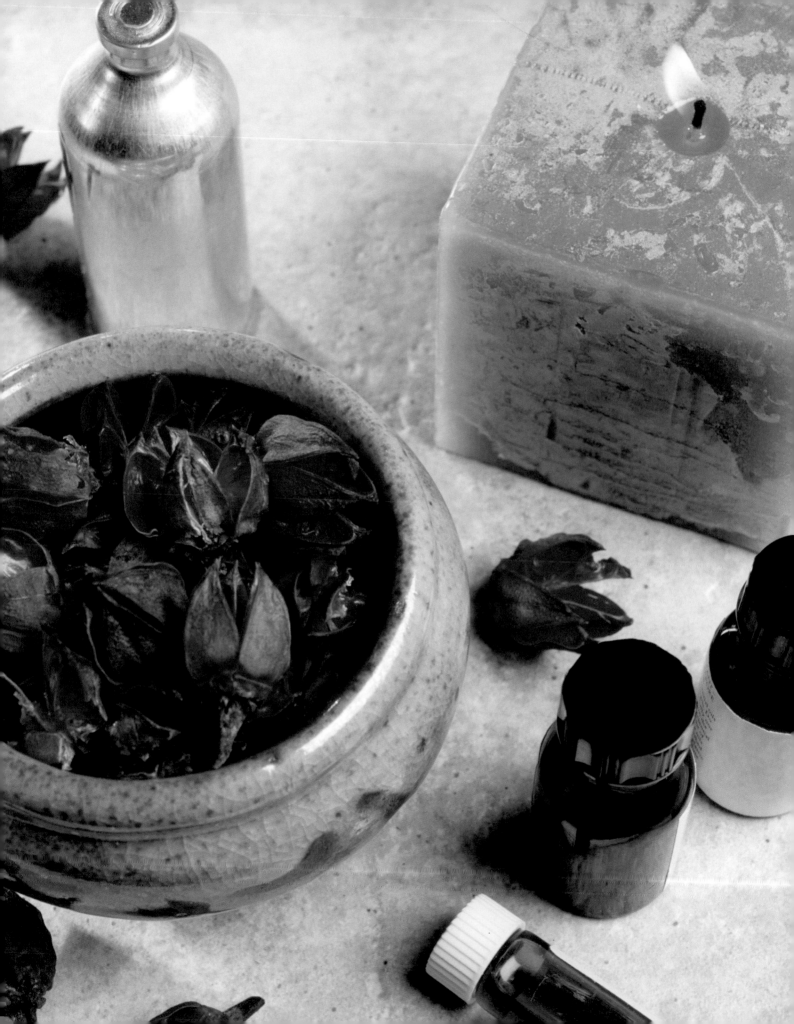

chapter two

using essential oils

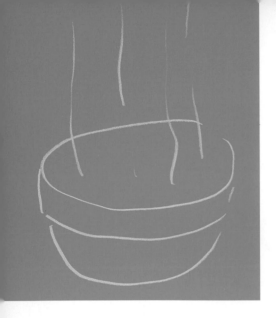

using essential oils

There are many ways to enjoy the healing benefits of aromatherapy and you will have lots of fun learning about and experimenting with some of the most popular methods outlined in this section. Be prepared to be creative and discover your own ways to bring aromatherapy into your daily life. You can create a beautiful aromatic environment whilst preventing and healing a multitude of common ailments. Enjoy!

aromatic baths

Mankind has employed aromatic baths throughout history for pleasure, rituals and healing. The Egyptians were experts in their use, and the Greeks and Romans used them extensively. Hippocrates, the 'Father of Medicine', claimed, 'The way to health is to have an aromatic bath and a scented massage every day'.

When we use essential oils in the bath, they are able to penetrate the skin due to their tiny molecular structure. In addition, as they evaporate we inhale them.

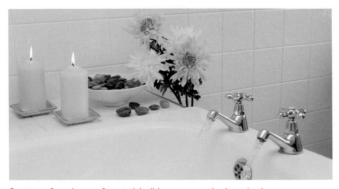

Scatter a few drops of essential oil into a warm bath and relax.

method

1. Shut the bathroom door.
2. Fill up the bath.
3. Scatter six drops of essential oil into the water. (NB Add them at the last moment as they evaporate quickly).
4. Disperse the oils as much as possible.
5. Stay in the bath for about 20 minutes (or longer if you really want to indulge!) to enjoy the full benefits of the essential oils.

using carrier oils in the bath

Essential oils are only partially soluble in water and can be diluted by adding them to a carrier oil (see pages 36–42). Mix six drops of essential oil in a tablespoon of a carrier oil such as sweet almond oil for a moisturising bath. You may also use milk, honey or a bath salt mixture as a carrier.

Specialist aromatherapy suppliers sell unscented foam bath and luxurious bath oil bases to help to disperse the essential oils. (See useful addresses on page 125.)

recipes

the de-stresser

To counteract anxiety and tension.

Lavender	2 drops
Chamomile	2 drops
Bergamot	2 drops

Relax in a warm bath, with dim lights and candles.

Take deep relaxing breaths.

the sleep inducer

Clary Sage	2 drops
Sandalwood	2 drops
Chamomile	2 drops

Indulge yourself in a long, hot, warm bath just before going to bed and enjoy your best night's sleep ever!

the revitaliser

Lemon	2 drops
Black pepper	2 drops
Rosemary	2 drops

An excellent to wake you up in the morning or to rejuvenate yourself after a long day at work ready for the evening.

the aches and pains buster

Frankincense	2 drops
Lavender	2 drops
Marjoram	2 drops

Soak in a long, warm bath after over exercising to relieve pain and soothe those aching muscles.

the night of passion

Jasmine	1 drop
Rose	1 drop
Sandalwood	2 drops
Ylang Ylang	2 drops

A wonderful aphrodisiac blend for you and your lover.

Burn some candles and play some soft music.

the big detox

1 teaspoon baking soda

2 teaspoons sea salt

4 teaspoons Epsom salts

Mix well, add the essential oils to the mixture and then add to the bath water.

Juniper	2 drops
Cypress	2 drops
Lemon	2 drops

A great blend for drawing out and eliminating those toxins!

the moisturiser

Sandalwood	2 drops
Carrot seed	3 drops
Rose	1 drop

Substitute geranium or palmarosa for rose if rose is too costly.

Add your essential oil to ¼ cup of goat's milk and then add to your bath.

Ideal for skin dried by exposure to the sun or in the winter.

the cellulite buster

Juniper	2 drops
Fennel	2 drops
Lemon	2 drops

Prior to bathing, perform dry brushing or use a loofah while bathing to encourage unsightly cellulite to disappear.

the colds and flu reliever

Cajeput	2 drops
Lavender	2 drops
Tea tree	2 drops

Inhale these scents in a warm bath to loosen mucus and boost your immune system – and get an early night to speed up your recovery.

the hormone balancer

Geranium	3 drops
Cypress	2 drops
Rose	1 drop

(You may substitute chamomile for rose if it is too expensive).

Great for P.M.T. and the menopause.

This formula really helps to regulate the hormones.

showers

If you do not have a bath, or are in a hurry to get to work, a shower is a quick and convenient way to enjoy the benefits of aromatherapy. Showers are a wonderful opportunity to wake you up. There are several ways of using essential oils in the shower.

method 1

1. Shut the bathroom door and shower door if you have one. Sprinkle no more than six drops of essential oil onto a sponge, flannel, soft mitt or other suitable cloth.
2. Massage your entire body gently with your blend of essential oils, and shower as usual. The oils will be absorbed through the skin and also via inhalation.

CAUTION
Never exceed six drops or you could irritate the skin. Do not use this method on broken or irritated skin.

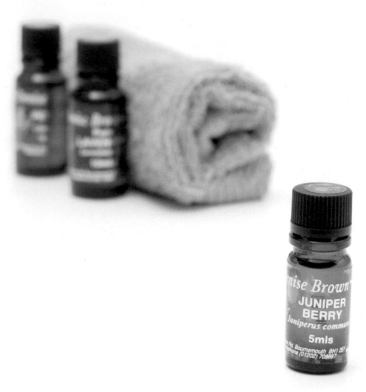
Sprinkle a few drops of essential oil on to a sponge or flannel for use in the shower.

method 2

1. Shut the bathroom door and shower as usual.
2. Almost at the end of your shower apply six drops of essential oil to your soft washcloth and rub all over your body.
3. Pat yourself dry very gently after your shower.

for sleek skin
If you wish, you may blend six drops of essential oil with a tablespoon of carrier oil. This will make your skin feel soft, nourished and supple, and is extremely beneficial for dry or ageing skin.

method 3

1. Close the bathroom door to keep in the precious aromas.
2. Plug the tray of your shower, turn on the water and add six drops of essential oil to the water. You will absorb the oils through your feet and as the vapours rise you will be surrounded by a sensuous-smelling mist.
Aromatherapy suppliers will stock special shower gels and unscented bath oils to which you can add your chosen essential oils. Try out any of the recipes in the previous bath section or create your own special formulae.

to boost circulation
Just before finishing your shower, turn on the cold water. This helps to stimulate a poor circulation and will make you feel refreshed and energised.

footbaths and hand baths

Footbaths and hand baths are a simple and highly effective way of using essential oils. You may not have the time for a shower or bath, or you may feel too lethargic to undress. For the elderly or those who have a disability, foot and hand baths are the ideal way to administer essential oils. Although only the hands or feet are submerged, the aromatics are effectively absorbed and the whole body is treated.

There is no excuse for not having the time for aromatherapy. You can enjoy a footbath while reading, studying or writing letters, and a hand bath may be experienced whilst watching your favourite television programme.

footbath method

Footbaths are great after standing on your feet all day at work. Runners and other athletes quickly become addicted to an aromatherapy foot soak which will rapidly relieve conditions such as athlete's foot and ease pain and swelling in the foot and ankles. Their power is hugely underestimated.

1. Fill a bowl half full of warm water.
2. Add six drops of your selected essential oils or essential oil blend.
3. Sit comfortably, plunge your feet into the therapeutic aromatic essences and soak for about 10–15 minutes. You may soak your feet for longer if you wish, but you will probably need to change the water as it becomes cold.
4. Pat your feet gently dry with your towel. For a real treat, massage your feet afterwards with an aromatherapy massage oil or cream (see page 35 for how to make a massage blend).

recipes

feel-good feet

Peppermint	3 drops
Lavender	2 drops
Chamomile	1 drop

This recipe is fantastic for soothing and cooling aching feet. Immerse your feet for about 10–15 minutes for immediate relief.

athlete's foot

Lavender	2 drops
Myrrh	2 drops
Tea tree	2 drops

Athlete's foot is an itchy, infectious condition that lurks between the toes. It loves warm, moist conditions such as changing rooms. Soak your feet daily with the above blend. If you wish, you may also dab neat tea tree or lavender onto the affected areas for faster results. Always wear cotton socks, dry your feet properly and make sure you don't share your towel with anyone.

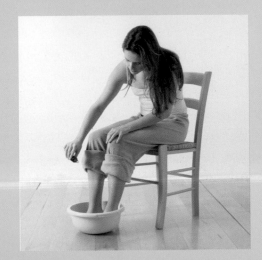

hand bath method

Hand baths are highly effective in relieving pain and swelling in the hands and are recommended for all conditions affecting the hands, such as arthritis, carpal tunnel syndrome, dermatitis and poor circulation. Anyone who uses their hands extensively such as hairdressers, gardeners, or computer personnel should have regular hand baths.

1. Fill one bowl or two smaller bowls half full of warm water.

2. Add six drops of your selected essential oil and/or carrier. Our hands can become very dry and rough, and a tablespoon of carrier oil is excellent for keeping the hands soft and supple.

3. Make yourself comfortable and if you are using a single bowl place it on your lap; if you are using two bowls place them on either side of you. Plunge your hands into the hand bath(s) for about 10–15 minutes and enjoy the beneficial properties of the essential oils.

4. Gently dry your hands and if you wish, massage them with a blend of oils you have previously prepared. (See page 35 for how to mix a massage blend.)

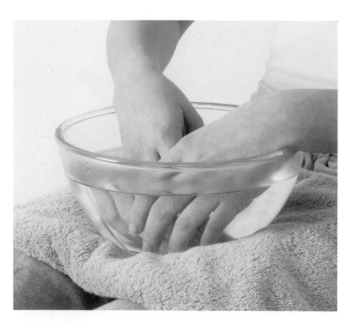

recipes

happy hands

Benzoin	2 drops
Chamomile	2 drops
Sandalwood	2 drops

This recipe helps to counteract dryness, soothes irritation and leaves hands soft and supple.

circulation booster

Black pepper	2 drops
Geranium	2 drops
Ginger	2 drops

Excellent for the winter months, this recipe dilates the capillaries, and increases the circulation to the hands.

arthritis blend

Lavender	2 drops
Frankincense	1 drop
Juniper	1 drop
Marjoram	2 drops

Regular hand baths can relieve pain, reduce inflammation, detoxify and increase mobility.

sitz baths / hip baths

A Sitz bath which literally means 'to sit' is an invaluable way to relieve all conditions affecting the perineal area. Problems such as cystitis, thrush, haemorrhoids, vaginal and anal itching and postnatal stitches or bruising, all respond remarkably well to a soak in a sitz bath.

hip baths
method

1. Fill a bidet, bath or a bowl that is large enough for you to sit in up to hip level with warm water.
2. Add four to six drops of your chosen essential oils and disperse thoroughly.
3. Sit in the bath for approximately ten minutes.
NB In order to clear a condition speedily, a hip bath should be taken two or three times daily for several days until the problem has cleared up.

sitz bath (alternate hot and cold method)

The alternate hot and cold sitz bath is employed by many naturopaths and in the more medically orientated health farms.

method

1. Find two bowls, both large enough for you to sit in, and fill one with tolerably hot water and the other with cold water.
2. Add four to six drops of your selected essential oils to each bowl and agitate thoroughly to disperse the oil.
3. Sit in the hot bath and at the same time put your feet in the cold bath. Remain there for about one minute.
4. Now change over. Sit in the cold bath (quite a shock if you haven't done this before!) and put your feet in the hot bath and stay there for about a minute.
5. Repeat the cycle two or three times. Carry out sitz baths twice daily for a few days until the condition has cleared up.

recipes

cystitis soother
Bergamot	2 drops
Juniper	2 drops
Sandalwood	2 drops

Sit in the bidet or a large bowl of warm water to which you have added your essential oils. To enhance the aromatic potion, mix the essential oils with one or two tablespoons of honey. This blend will provide soothing and healing relief and will fight off bacteria. After washing, pat the area gently dry with a soft cotton towel.

haemorrhoid reliever
Cypress	2 drops
Geranium	2 drops
Myrrh	2 drops

This recipe helps to prevent haemorrhoids from forming and will shrink them down, relieving the pain, itching, swelling and bleeding. Make sure you increase your dietary roughage to avoid constipation and the resultant straining that leads to constipation. Increase fluids, avoid sitting for too long and take regular exercise.

after stitches repairer
Chamomile	2 drops
Lavender	2 drops
Tea tree	2 drops

This aromatherapy sitz bath will increase the rate of healing, provide pain relief, soothe inflammation and prevent and fight off any infection.

compresses

A compress is an excellent way to treat muscular aches and pains, bruises, sprains and strains, fevers and headaches.

Compresses may be applied either hot or cold and it is important to know which is appropriate.

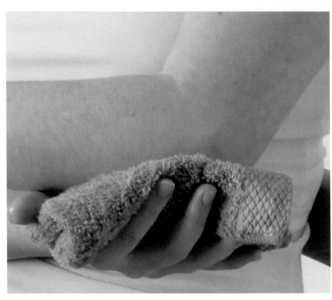

Use an aromatic compress to soothe away aches and pains.

cold compress

Use for hot swellings and inflammations, such as a sprained ankle or an inflamed knee. Also for fevers, headaches and any recent acute injury.

method

1. Fill a small bowl with very cold, preferably icy water.
2. Add six drops of your chosen essential oils.
3. Soak a flannel, small towel or piece of cotton fabric in the water.
4. Wring out the excess and place the compress over the area to be treated if necessary.
5. Cover with a piece of clingfilm and a bandage to keep it in place. For extra cooling power, place an ice pack on top.
6. When the compress becomes warm it may be replaced with a cold one.

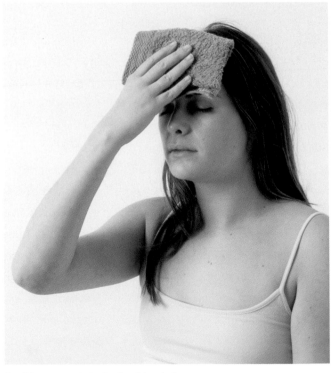

A cold compress helps to dispell headaches.

hot compress

Use for old injuries, or for treating chronic long-term pain and for drawing out pus from boils.

method

1. Fill a small bowl with water as hot as you can comfortably bear.
2. Add six drops of essential oil.
3. Place a flannel, small towel or piece of natural fabric in the hot aromatic water.
4. Wring out any excess water, apply it to the affected area and if necessary, secure it with clingfilm and a bandage. The compress may be renewed once it has cooled down to body temperature. Compresses may be applied several times a day as and whenever necessary.

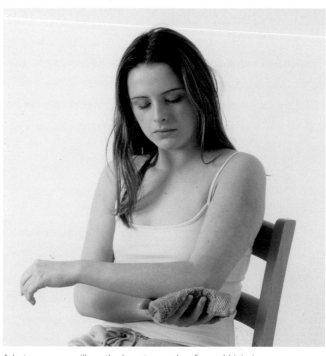

A hot compress will soothe long-term aches from old injuries.

recipes

inflammation subsider

cold compress

Chamomile	2 drops
Cypress	2 drops
Geranium	1 drop
Rosemary	1 drop

This recipe is excellent for a sprained joint, a pulled muscle, or any sports or other injury. The injured part should be rested and elevated to accelerate the healing process.

fever reducer

cold compress

Chamomile	2 drops
Lavender	2 drops
Peppermint	2 drops

Cold compresses are a tried and tested method for bringing down a high fever. Place the compress either on the forehead or on the back of the neck. A fresh compress should be reapplied once it reaches body temperature. If the fever rises above 103°F then call the doctor.

chronic pain reliever

hot compress

Black pepper	2 drops
Ginger	1 drop
Marjoram	2 drops
Juniper	1 drop

This method is excellent for easing the discomfort of arthritis and rheumatism, or indeed any old injury or chronic long term pain. Do not use a hot compress over inflamed and swollen areas as this will induce pain and possibly tissue damage – a cold compress is indicated in these circumstances.

gargles and mouthwashes

Gargles are extremely helpful for conditions such as sore throats, laryngitis and loss of voice.

Mouthwashes are an excellent way to sweeten the breath and to treat and prevent problems such as mouth ulcers and gum disorders.

method 1 quick and easy

1. Put two teaspoons of apple cider vinegar (preferably organic) in a small glass.
2. Add two drops of your chosen essential oil(s) and stir well. Essential oils dissolve slightly better in vinegar than in water, and cider vinegar is a well-known remedy for the throat.
3. Fill the glass with warm water.
4. Gargle two to three times daily.

N.B. If you do not have any cider vinegar then just add your essential oils to a glass of warm water.

method 2

1. In a glass or cup add your essential oils to a teaspoon of honey.
2. Make some chamomile or sage herbal tea and add half a cup to the honey mixture until it is dissolved.
3. If you wish, add a teaspoon of fresh lemon juice and/or a teaspoon of apple cider vinegar.
4. Top up your cup, stir well and gargle. Do not swallow the gargle and try not to eat or drink anything immediately after gargling. It is best to wait about 20 minutes to enable the essential oils to be absorbed.

N.B. The honey in this recipe acts as a carrier for the oils, has anti-inflammatory and anti-bacterial properties and is renowned for its soothing action on the throat – many throat lozenges contain honey. Fresh lemon juice is a powerful anti-bacterial agent and is excellent for detoxification and counteracting acid. Apple cider vinegar is medicinal and extremely beneficial and is a classic remedy for sore throats.

recipes

sore throat soother

Geranium	1 drop
Lemon	1 drop

Use these oils in either method 1 or 2. This recipe will help to fight the infection, decrease the inflammation and soothe the rough and raw sensations of the sore throat. If the sore throat persists for several days, it is advisable to seek the advice of a medically qualified doctor.

mouth ulcer buster

Myrrh	1 drop
Tea tree	1 drop

Incorporate these oils in either method 1 or 2 to banish mouth ulcers. The recipe will help to alleviate pain and will accelerate healing time. If you use this remedy on a regular basis you will find that the number of attacks will decrease dramatically and eventually stop.

sweet breath

Peppermint or Fennel	1 drop
Lemon	1 drop

Use this recipe daily after brushing your teeth to prevent and combat bad breath. Your mouth will tingle with freshness and you family and friends will really appreciate it!

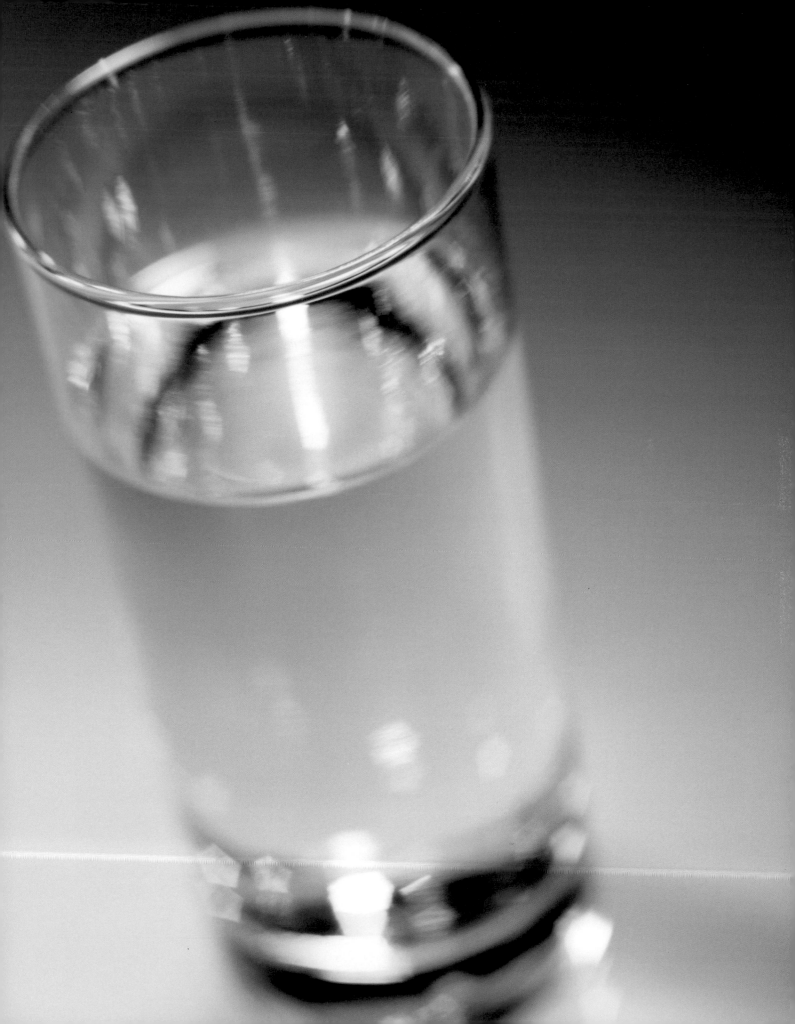

inhalations

Inhalations are not, as you might imagine, just for relieving the symptoms of coughs, colds and sinusitis. They affect not only the body, but also the mind and even the spirit.

Inhalations can be used to counteract stress and anxiety, lift the mood, stimulate clarity of thought and boost the memory. Essential oils can positively enhance our home and office environments. They purify the air, provide natural fragrance and make us feel wonderful.

They are also a very powerful meditation aid, opening us up to other levels of awareness. For centuries aromatics have been burnt in religious ceremonies and for purification rites. The Latin *per fumum* (the derivation of the word 'perfume') means 'through smoke'.

You can use oils such as lemon and rosemary in the morning to help to wake you up and a blend of sandalwood and lavender in the evening to assist relaxation.

There are a wide variety of methods used for inhalation. We will explore some of these:

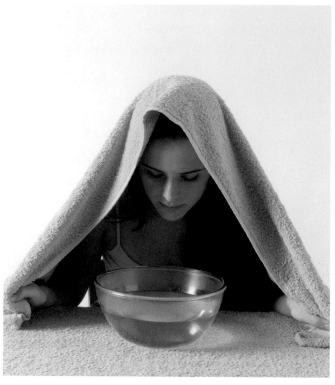

Inhale the vapours of essential oils to tackle stress and aid relaxation.

steam inhalation

An excellent method for the respiratory system to ease nasal and chest congestion. Steaming is also excellent for cleansing the skin.

method

1. Pour near-boiling water into a glass or ceramic bowl.
2. Add two to four drops of essential oil.
3. Cover your head with a towel and lean over the bowl to form a 'tent'.
4. Keep your eyes closed and breathe slowly and deeply inhaling the therapeutic aromatic steam. Stay there for about five minutes to obtain maximum benefit.
If you are suffering from a cold or the flu you may take steam inhalation two to three times daily.

recipe

cold reliever

Cajeput	1 drop
Lemon	1 drop
Rosemary	1 drop

This recipe provides a powerful decongestant for the respiratory tract. Use it for coughs, colds and flu to loosen mucus and speed up recovery.

handkerchief
method

Sprinkle a few drops of essential oil onto a handkerchief, tissue or cotton wool ball and inhale as required.

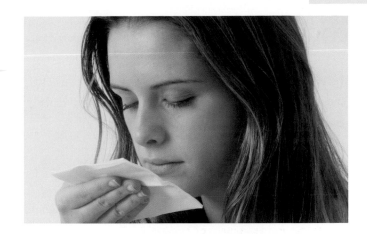

hands
method

Place just one drop of essential oil onto your palm and rub your hands together briskly. Cup your hands over your nose and inhale the aroma deeply until you feel relaxed.
The 'hand method' is particularly effective for acute distress in a crisis situation such as a panic attack. Sufferers should carry a small plastic bottle of lavender or chamomile in their pocket or on their person to alleviate attacks.

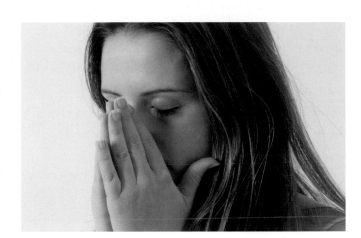

pillow
method

Sprinkle a few drops of essential oil onto your pillow, or alternatively, onto a piece of cotton wool and place it inside your pillowcase.
The 'pillow method' is a wonderful way to enjoy a peaceful night's sleep. Try chamomile, marjoram, sandalwood or lavender.

recipes

If you have a cold or sinusitis, try eucalyptus, cajeput, myrtle or rosemary to clear the nasal passages. Sufferers from motion sickness should sprinkle a few drops of ginger, peppermint or spearmint onto a handkerchief and inhale deeply while in the car, boat, or plane.

room fragrancing

light bulb ring

These fragrance rings, which are usually ceramic or metal, fit on to a light bulb.

method

Simply sprinkle a few drops of essential oil onto the ring and the warmth from the bulb will release the healing vapours.

Since essential oils are flammable be cautious – only apply the oils when the ring is cold. Also, if you wash the ring after use dry it thoroughly to avoid a electric shock!

room mist spray

Room mists are a wonderful way to deliciously scent your home, change the mood or to purify the atmosphere.

method

Add 10–15 drops of essential oil to a small house plant spray filled with water. Shake the bottle thoroughly and then spray around the room.

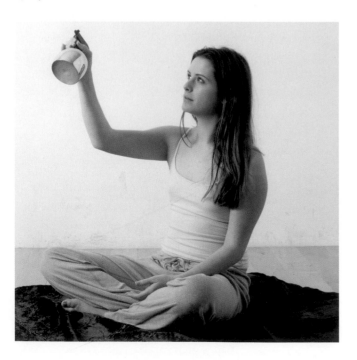

recipes

N.B. Add the drops to a small house plant spray filled with water.

bust those bugs

Tea tree	5 drops
Thyme	5 drops
Lemon	5 drops

The antiseptic properties of these three potent oils will soon disinfect a room at home or in the workplace and kill off germs.

lovers' mist

Rose	2 drops
Jasmine	4 drops
Sandalwood	5 drops

This is a great aphrodisiac! Lightly spray your bedroom, bed linen, nightwear or yourself to encourage a night of passion.

banish odours

Lemongrass	5 drops
Juniper	5 drops
Pine	5 drops

A highly effective blend for neutralising stale cooking odours and combating the lingering smell of cigarette smoke and paint. A must for after a party!

candles

The majority of the so-called 'aromatherapy' candles on sale are perfumed with synthetic aromas. It is far better to make your own and so simple!

method

Light a candle and leave it until the wax starts to melt. Blow it out and add one to two drops of essential oil onto the melted wax. Relight the candle and allow the beautiful aromas to permeate the room.

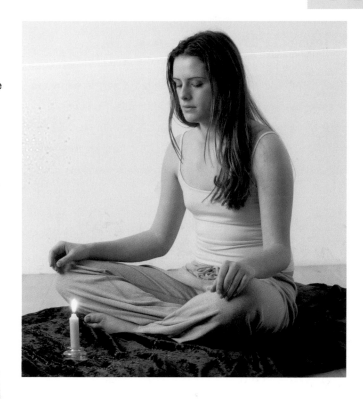

vaporisation

1. simple oil burner

The cheapest and most readily available oil burners are made of earthenware. A nightlight candle is used as the heat source and is placed inside the burner under a small bowl (that may be detachable) that is filled with water. Sprinkle a few drops of essential oil into the water and as it heats up the aroma will gently perfume the air. For faster results, fill the bowl with hot rather than cold water, otherwise the candle has to heat the water and the process will be slower. Do make sure that you keep the water topped up in the bowl. When buying a vaporiser choose one with a deep reservoir.

Ideal essential oils to use as insect repellents include citronella, basil, cajeput, cedarwood, rosemary, peppermint, eucalyptus, geranium, juniper, lemongrass and tea tree.

2. electric diffuser

A more expensive modern high-tech devise is the electric diffuser. These are appropriate for diffusing essential oils into offices, health clubs, hospitals and so on. The single clay burner already described is more than sufficient for home use.

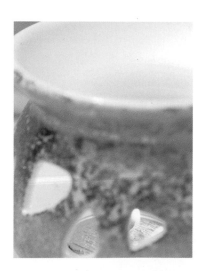

massage

An aromatherapy massage is a wonderful way to enjoy the healing, therapeutic effects of essential oils. However, it must be remembered that essential oils should NEVER be applied to the skin undiluted in their neat form as they are highly concentrated and are likely to irritate the skin.

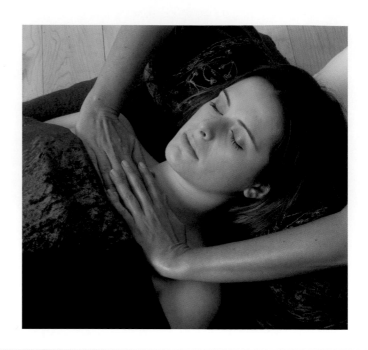

vegetable NOT mineral

Pure essential oils are diluted in a natural 'base' oil otherwise known as a 'carrier' oil. Vegetable, nut or seed oils are most appropriate since they contain vitamins, minerals and essential fatty acids all of which are very beneficial to the skin. Mineral oil (often marketed as baby oil) is not suitable for aromatherapy. It is a refined oil popular in many commercial products since it is inexpensive and has an indefinite shelf life. However, it has a large molecular structure and not only prevents nutrients and essential oils from entering the skin, it also hinders the excretion of waste through the pores. It does not moisturise the skin (as the advertisements claim) – it dries and clogs the skin, encouraging the development of blackheads and pimples.

unrefined NOT refined

Refined oils are not suitable for use in aromatherapy. Most oils that you find on supermarket shelves will be refined and contain preservatives to prolong their shelf life as well as artificial colours to make them more attractive to the consumer! Although refined oil will not usually harm the skin it is not therapeutic.

cold-pressed NOT solvent-extracted

Cold-pressed oils are the most suitable for use in aromatherapy. These oils have been pressed – chemical solvents have not been used to extract them. Oils produced via hot extraction may be less expensive as a higher yield is produced, but they are of an inferior quality. You do get what you pay for, so expect to pay more for high quality cold-pressed oils.

To sum up, carrier oils should be **cold-pressed, unrefined** and **vegetable.**

mixing massage oils

When blending essential oils with a carrier oil, the dilution is usually between 0.5% and 3%. The lowest concentrations are useful for children and those with highly sensitive skin. Many aromatherapists do not use a concentration above 2%.

The following information explains just what a 1%, 2% dilution, etc. really is.

0.5% = 1 drop of essential oil diluted in 10 ml base oil
1%   = 1 drop of essential oil diluted in 5 ml base oil
2%   = 2 drops of essential oil diluted in 5 ml base oil
3%   = 3 drops of essential oil diluted in 5 ml base oil

To make this clearer:
5 ml   = one teaspoon   = 100 drops
10 ml = two teaspoons = 200 drops

For general blending purposes, I suggest you follow these simple guidelines:

Add 3 drops of essential oil to 10 ml (2 teaspoons) carrier oil.
6 drops of essential oil to 20 ml carrier oil
15 drops of essential oil to 50 ml carrier oil
30 drops of essential oil to 100 ml carrier oil

If you are treating a small area of the body 10 ml will be ample. For a complete massage, mix up 20 ml. Remember, if you are making up a larger quantity for storing them, you must use amber-coloured glass bottles.

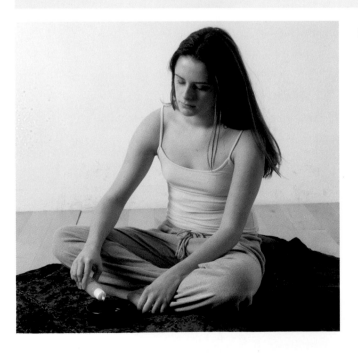

mixing tips

- Work in a well-lit, well-ventilated area.
- Do not blend on polished or plastic surfaces as. accidental spills of essential oils can cause damage.
- Double check the essential oil(s) you are using and the dilution amount.
- Measure out the carrier oil.
- Add the drops of essential oil.
- If you are making up a blend to keep, store it in an amber-coloured glass bottle and label the contents and put a date on it.
- Wipe up any spills to avoid damage to any surfaces.
- Wash your hands thoroughly afterwards, as neat essential oils can irritate the eyes and skin.
- Store your oils properly as detailed on page 15.

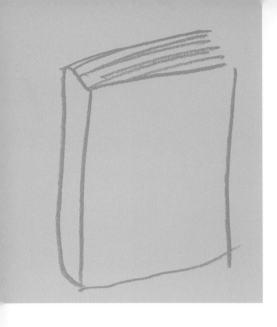

a directory of carrier oils

key

Use this simple key to identify the uses for each carrier oil.

 Suitable for all skin types.

 Suitable for dry skin.

 Excellent moisturiser.

 Suitable for elderly/aged skin.

 Suitable for inflamed or broken skin.

 Sun-damaged skin.

 Suitable for delicate or sensitive skin.

 Suitable for itchy skin.

 Suitable for greasy skin.

almond oil (sweet)
prunus amygdalis

description: A light, pale yellow oil with a delicate aroma that is widely used in aromatherapy. Sweet almond oil is possibly the most popular carrier oil and is widely available.

uses:

· All types of skin

· Itchy skin conditions

· Dry skin

· Sensitive skin

· Prematurely aged skin

percentage in blends: 100%: can be used as a base oil.

availability

Widely available from health shops and chemists, but make sure it is not refined.

apricot kernel
prunus armenica

description: A very light, finely textured oil that is readily absorbed by the skin.

uses:

· All types of skin

· Prematurely aged skin

· Delicate, sensitive skin

· Inflamed skin

· Dry skin

percentage in blends: 100%: can be used as a base oil.

availability: Obtainable from some health shops and by mail order from aromatherapy specialists.

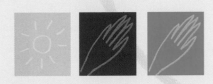

avocado oil
prunus americana

description: Avocado is cold-pressed from the flesh and has a sludgy dark green appearance – a good sign that it has not been refined. If you see pale yellow avocado oil it has been refined and is therefore lacking in nutrients.

uses:

· Excellent penetrative powers

· Dry skin

· Wrinkles

· Sun damaged skin

· Prematurely aged skin

percentage in blends: Usually added to a blend (up to 25%).

availability: For good quality, unrefined avocado oil you will need a reliable essential oil supplier.

calendula oil
calendula officinalis

description: Otherwise known as marigold oil, calendula is an 'infused' or 'macerated' oil. This means that the fresh plant material (ie marigolds) has been chopped up, placed into a vat of vegetable oil such as virgin olive oil and agitated over a period of time.

uses:

· Cracked and chapped skin
· Sore and inflamed skin
· Burns
· Chillblains
· Itchy skin
· Eczema
· Bed sores
· Broken veins
· Varicose veins
· Nappy rash
· Cracked nipples

percentage in blends: May be used on its own but it is usually added to an aromatherapy blend (up to 25%). Calendula oil is sometimes blended 50/50 with St John's Wort Oil (hypericum) – see later entry.

availability: Obtainable from essential oil suppliers, or you can try making your own.

recipe for calendula oil

1. Half-fill a large screw top glass jar with with chopped-up plant material.
2. Cover the marigold material with virgin olive oil (preferably warm).
3. Shake thoroughly.
4. Place the container in a warm place, on a sunny window sill or even outside in the sun for at least one week. (Bring it in at night). Make sure that you agitate it daily.
5. When the oil is ready, filter off the plant material by straining it through a piece of muslin or a fine nylon sieve. Bottle your oil and label. If you wish you may add a small amount of wheatgerm oil which is high in vitamin E (a natural antioxidant).

corn oil
zea mays

description: Obtained from sweet corn kernels, it is a yellow oil with a faint characteristic corn-on-the-cob colour.

uses:

All skin types

percentage in blends: 100%: can be used as a base oil.

availability: Obtainable from some aromatherapy suppliers. Take care not to buy the refined oil which is used for cooking.

grapeseed oil
vitis vinifera

description: A virtually colourless, odourless carrier oil with a very fine texture. This makes it a popular choice with some aromatherapists, although personally I do not favour carrier oil produced by hot extraction.

uses:
· All skin types
· Oily skin

percentage in blends: 100%: can be used as a base oil, although most aromatherapists prefer to add other carrier oils to it.

availability: Widely available and inexpensive.

evening primrose oil
oenorthera biennis

description: A relatively expensive oil with a very fine texture extracted from the seeds. It contains GLA (Gamma Linolenic Acid) and is widely used in capsule form as a nutritional supplement to combat conditions such as PMS, eczema, heart disease, multiple sclerosis, arthritis, and allergies.

uses:
· Eczema
· Allergic skin
· Psoriasis
· Dermatitis
· Ageing skin
· Dry skin

percentage in blends: A small amount is usually added to a blend in approximately a 10% dilution. You may break open a couple of capsules and add to your blend.

availability: Capsules are widely available. The oil is best obtained from aromatherapy specialists.

hypericum / st john's wort
hypericum perforatum

description: St John's Wort, like calendula, is a 'macerated' or 'infused' oil made from the flowering tops that impart a ruby red colour to the oil.

uses:
· Inflamed skin
· Sunburn
· Muscle and joint pain
· Inflamed nerves

percentage in blends: St John's Wort is usually added to a blend and may be mixed 50/50 with calendula oil.

availability: Obtainable from specialist suppliers.

Caution! Excessive use of St John's Wort may cause a skin allergy in hypersensitive individuals which can become aggravated on exposure to sunlight.

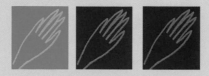

olive oil
olea europaea

description: A green oil available in different grades. Always use cold-pressed extra virgin or virgin olive oil.

uses:

· Inflamed skin

· Rheumatic skin

· Itchy skin

· Dry, dehydrated skin

· Dry and brittle hair

(Taken internally it is useful for constipation and to protect against heart disease.)

percentage in blends: As it is rather heavy and has a distinctive aroma, olive oil is normally diluted 50/50 with a less viscous oil such as sweet almond.

availability: Widely available from supermarkets.

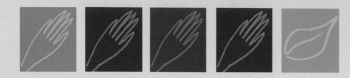

jojoba oil
simmondsia chinensis

description: A light yellow oil that is virtually odourless, it is extremely stable and therefore has good keeping qualities. Although it is one of the more expensive oils it makes an excellent facial and hair oil.

uses:

· All skin types

· Excellent moisturiser

· Unclogs the pores

· Oily skin

· Acne

· Dry skin

· Inflamed skin

· Eczema

· Hair care

percentage in blends: 100% Jojoba may be used, although it is usually added to a blend.

availability: Good-quality jojoba oil can be obtained from aromatherapy suppliers.

safflower oil
carthamus tinctorius

description: A yellow oil with a faint nutty aroma that is not very stable and is therefore prone to oxidation.

uses:

· All skin types

· Inflamed skin

percentage in blends: Can be used as a base oil 100%.

availability: Refined safflower oil is available from some supermarkets. The unrefined oil which is, of course, preferable, is available from aromatherapy suppliers.

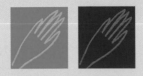

sesame oil
sesamum indicum

description: A pale yellow oil when it is cold pressed, with a slightly nutty aroma. Sesame is widely used in Ayurvedic medicine in India.

uses:

· All skin types

· Dry skin

· Eczema

· Psoriasis

· Protects against the sun. Sesame oil has a sunscreen factor of SPF 4.

percentage in blends: 100%: can be used as a base oil.

availability: Do not use the strongly flavoured, dark brown oil used in Chinese cooking. Good quality oil is obtainable from reputable aromatherapy suppliers.

sunflower oil
helianthus annus

description: A yellow oil with a slightly detectable nutty aroma and a light texture.

uses:

· All skin types

percentage in blends: 100%: can be used as a base oil.

availability: Refined oil is available from supermarkets. Unrefined oil is obtainable from health food shops.

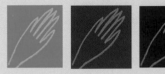

wheatgerm oil
triticum vulgare

description: A natural antioxidant, wheatgerm oil is a heavy orangey-brown oil with a distinctive odour.

uses:

· Dry, cracked skin

· Itchy skin

· Eczema

· Mature skin

· Repairs damage caused by too much sun

· Varicose veins

· Heals scars

· Stretchmarks

percentage in blends: Use up to a 10% dilution as wheatgerm is too thick and sticky to use on its own for massage. A small amount is often added to blends to increase the keeping qualities.

availability: Cold-pressed wheatgerm oil can be obtained from aromatherapy suppliers.

other carrier oils in brief

borage seed oil
borago officinalis

An expensive oil usually added to aromatherapy blends to regenerate skin cells. Also known as 'starflower oil', it is taken as a nutritional supplement.

carrot oil
daucus carota

A macerated oil not to be confused with the essential oil. Carrot oil is usually added in up to a 10% dilution for its anti-ageing and skin rejuvenating properties.

castor oil
ricinus communis

A heavy, sticky oil not really suitable for massage purposes. Castor oil is used in protective skin and hair products, such as conditioners and nappy rash creams. It has also been recommended for various cutaneous complaints, such as ringworm, itch, etc.

coconut oil
cocus nucifera

A highly refined oil with a distinctive aroma that is solid at room temperature. It aids sun tanning and is used in skin and hair products. However, it may cause a rash on hypersensitive skin. In the past it was a popular massage oil, but more suitable oils have become widely available.

hazelnut oil
corylus avellana

Hazelnut oil has a nutty aroma and is very penetrative with a slightly astringent action. It is usually diluted 50/50 with another carrier oil such as sweet almond and is beneficial for oily skin and acne.

macadamia oil
macadamia integrifolia

A relatively new arrival on the aromatherapy scene from Australia, macadamia oil is golden with a light texture when unrefined. It is useful for dry and mature skin, as well as sunburn.

passiflora oil
passiflora incarnata

Available in capsules which can pierced and added to a blend to promote the elasticity of the skin.

peach kernel oil
prunus persica

A very light, finely textured oil that is readily absorbed by the skin.

peanut oil
arachnis hypogaea

Peanut oil has a nutty aroma and a sticky texture and is usually diluted with another carrier oil. It can be used for sunburn.

rosehip oil
rosa canina

A golden red oil that is very rejuvenating and healing. It can help scars, wounds, burns and aged skin.

soya bean oil
glycine soja

Suitable for all skin types, soya oil can be used as a base oil 100%. However, care should be taken with highly sensitive skins.

a directory of
essential oils

There are hundreds of aromatic oils available and space simply does not permit details of every known essential oil.

I have chosen 30 of the most common essential oils, selected for their wide range of benefits. Start off by buying just a few essential oils and gradually add to your collection. It is not necessary to buy them all at once — a great deal can be achieved with just a few essential oils.

key

Use this simple key to identify the properties of each essential oil.

 Decongestive.

 Aphrodisiac.

 Calming/soothing.

 Anti-depressant.

 Balancing

 Rejuvenating/ stimulant.

 Detoxifying.

 Digestive.

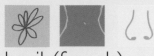

basil (french)
'the decongestive and restorer'

botanical name: *Ocimum basilicum*
aroma: Clear, fresh, sweet-spicy
properties: Uplifting -
Strengthening - Clarifying -
Decongestive
main uses
mind: A great tonic for the nerves
combating mental fatigue, anxiety and
depression.

body:

digestive
· Vomiting
· Stomach cramps
· Hiccups
· Cleanses the system
muscles/joints
· Muscle spasms e.g. cramp
· After exercise for tired muscles
· Strengthens muscles
· Headaches
reproductive
· Scanty and painful periods

respiratory
· Sinus problems
· Asthma
· Coughs and colds
· Restores sense of smell
skin
· Excellent insect repellent
blends well with: Bergamot,
geranium, lavender, neroli
contraindications:
· Avoid in pregnancy
· Take care with sensitive skin
price: Medium price range

bergamot
'the balancer'

botanical name: *Citrus bergamia*
aroma: Light, fresh, citrus
properties: Antidepressant -
Balancing - Uplifting
main uses
mind: Bergamot is renowned for its
ability to treat nervous tension, stress-
related disorders and depression.

body:

digestive
· Regulates
  appetite
· Eating disorders
· Colic
· Bad breath
reproductive
· Vaginal itching
· Vaginal
  discharges
· PMS

skin
· Acne
· Oily skin
· Cold sores
· Boils
· Chicken pox
· Eczema
· Insect repellent
urinary
· Infections such
  as cystitis

blends well with: All oils
especially neroli, chamomile, geranium
and cypress
contraindications:
· Do not apply prior to sunbathing as it
increases photosensitivity of the skin.
price: Medium price range

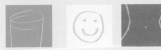

black pepper
'the warming tonic'

botanical name: *Piper nigrum*
aroma: Sharp, spicy, hot, warming
properties: Detoxifying - Stimulant - Tonic - Warming

main uses
mind: This is a real 'get-up-and-go' oil. It stimulates and strengthens the nerves, fills you with courage and stamina, and combats coldness and apathy.

body:
circulatory
· Poor circulation
· Anaemia
digestive
· Constipation
· Sluggish digestion
· Food poisoning
· Restores tone to the colon
· Loss of appetite

muscles/joints ·
All muscular aches and pains
· Rheumatism
· Arthritis
· Stiffness
· Before and after sport
respiratory
· Colds and flu
· Clears out mucous
· Chills

blends well with: Other spices, frankincense, geranium, rosemary
contraindications: None
price: Medium price range

cajeput
'the decongestive'

botanical name: *Melaleuca leucodendron*
aroma: Penetrating, camphorous, medicinal
properties: Decongestive - Stimulating - Warming

main uses
mind: Cajeput stimulates the mind, dispelling mental fatigue and lethargy.

body:
muscles/joints ·
Rheumatism
· Stiffness in joints
· Weakness
· Aches and pains
· Muscle fatigue
· Pain relief

respiratory
· All respiratory problems
· Sinusitis
· Colds and flu
· Bronchitis
· Throat problems
skin
· Lice
· Insect bites
· Chronic acne

blends well with: Bergamot, cypress, lemon, pine
contraindications:
· Use in a low dilution for those with sensitive skin.
price: Low-Medium price range

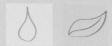

cedarwood atlas
'peace, harmony and tranquillity'

botanical name: *Cedrus atlantica*
aroma: Sweet, woody, warm
properties: Calming - Soothing - Sedative - Warming

main uses
mind: Cedarwood brings the mind back into balance, clearing away tension and anxiety. Excellent for meditation.

body:
respiratory
· Coughs and colds
· Catarrh
· Bronchitis
skin
· Acne
· Cellulite
· Dermatitis

· Fungal Infection
· Oily skin and hair
· Psoriasis
· Dandruff
· Eczema
urinary
· Cystitis
· Burning pains
· Itching

blends well with: Cypress, frankincense, neroli, rosewood
contraindications:
· Avoid during pregnancy
price: Medium price range

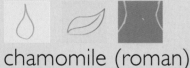

chamomile (roman)
'the BIG soother'

botanical name: Anthemis nobilis
aroma: Sweet, apple-like, aromatic, warm
properties: Balancing - Calming - Combats redness

main uses
mind: A remarkable oil for calming and soothing the mind, easing tension, anxiety, irritability, anger and restlessness. Frees the mind from worry ensuring a peaceful nights sleep. Relaxes children.

body:
digestive
· Colitis
· Gastritis
· Diarrhoea
· Vomiting
· Wind
· Irritable bowel syndrome
· Liver problems
muscles/joints · ·
· Aches and pains
· Headaches
· Arthritis
· Rheumatism

· Cramp
· Sprains and strains
· Neuralgia
· Toothache
reproductive
· Regulates menstruation
· Menopause
· Period pain
· PMS
skin
· Dry skin
· Sensitive skin
· Eczema
· Itching

· Allergies
· Acne
· Burns
· Inflamed skin
· Sores
· Blisters
· Psoriasis
urinary
· Cystitis
· Fluid retention

blends well with: Geranium, jasmine, neroli, palmarosa, rose
contraindications: None
price: High price range
N.B Do not buy Moroccan Chamomile

clary sage
'the ultimate euphoric'

botanical name: Salvia sclarea
aroma: Sweet, heady, floral
properties: Euphoric - Intoxicating - Tonic
main uses
mind: Clary sage will calm even the most overactive mind. It induces a sense of well-being and a 'couldn't-care-less' attitude. A must for all stress-related disorders.

body:
circulatory
· High blood pressure
muscles/joints
· Muscular tension
· Cramp
reproductive
· Tonic for the womb
· Infertility
· PMS
· Period pain
· Childbirth

respiratory
· Asthma
· Difficulty breathing due to tension
skin
· Inflamed skin
· Aged skin
· Wrinkles
· Sunburn
· Oily skin
· Allergic, hypersensitive skin

blends well with: Bergamot, frankincense, geranium, neroli, rose
contraindications:
· Avoid during pregnancy
· Do not use large doses and alcohol together
price: Medium price range

cypress
'the oil of change'

botanical name: Cupressus sempervirens
aroma: Woody, balsamic
properties: Astringent - Fluid reducing - Tonic
main uses
mind: Cypress is useful in times of change, e.g. moving house, changing career, forming new relationships or cutting old ties. It also helps to ease the sadness of bereavement. Cypress has a soothing effect on anger and irritability.

body:
circulatory
· Varicose veins
· Haemorrhoids
· Poor circulation
reproductive
· PMS
· Menopause
· Heavy periods
respiratory
· Whooping cough

· Asthma
· Flu
· Sore throat
skin
· Oily skin
· Acne
· Cellulite
· Broken capillaries
· Excessive perspiration

blends well with: Citrus oils, geranium, frankincense, juniper, neroli, rose
contraindications: None
price: Medium price range

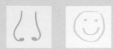

eucalyptus
'time to breathe'

botanical name: *Eucalyptus globulus*
aroma: Fresh, penetrating, cooling
properties: Expectorant - Stimulant
main uses
mind: Eucalyptus clears the head of mental exhaustion and increases our powers of concentration. It also cools down the emotions and gives us a 'breathing space'.
body:
muscles/joints · Pain relief
· Muscular aches
· Rheumatism
· Arthritis

· Fibrositis
· Neuralgia
· Congestive headaches
respiratory
· All respiratory problems
· Coughs and colds
· Flu
· Fevers
· Catarrh
· Sinusitis
· Throat problems

· Hay fever
· Bronchitis
· Boosts the immune system
skin
·Head lice
·Shingles
·Measles
·Herpes
·Chicken pox
·Wounds
·Blisters
·Stings

urinary
· Cystitis
· Fluid retention
blends well with: Bergamot, lavender, lemon, pine
contraindications:
· Do not massage on babies and young children
·Store away from homeopathic medicine
price: Low price range

fennel
'the big detox'

botanical name: *Foeniculum vulgare*
aroma: Aniseed-like, strong
properties: Detoxifying - Cleansing - Stimulating
main uses
mind: Fennel clears and enlivens the mind. It induces a sense of courage and strength and is a valuable asset when dieting, giving up smoking, etc.
body:
digestive
· Clears toxins
· Obesity

· Dieting
· Hangovers
· Tonic
· Indigestion
· Nausea
· Constipation
· Flatulence
· Halitosis (bad breath)
reproductive
· Regulates menstruation
· Menopause

· Promotes milk flow when breastfeeding
skin
· Cellulite
· Bruises
· Toxic, congested skin
urinary
· Fluid retention
· Clears waste

blends well with: Cypress, geranium, lemon, juniper, sandalwood
contraindications:
· Avoid during pregnancy
· Epileptics should avoid fennel
price: Medium price range

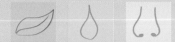

frankincense
'release, let go and move on'

botanical name: *Boswellia carterii*
aroma: Woody, spicy, balsamic
properties: Elevating - Healing - Rejuvenating

main uses

mind: An excellent aid for meditation, frankincense produces a heightened spiritual awareness. It enables us to release anxiety, tension and deep-seated problems from the past that may be impeding our progress.

body:

reproductive
· PMS
· Painful menstruation tonic

respiratory
· Slows down and deepens breathing
· Asthma

· Sinus congestion
· Laryngitis
· Bronchitis

skin
· Ageing skin
· Wrinkles
· Acne
· Scars
· Wounds
· Stretchmarks
· Haemorrhoids

blends well with: Citrus oils, cedarwood, rose, neroli, sandalwood
contraindications: None
price: Medium to high price range

geranium
'the hormone balancer'

botanical name: *Pelargonium graveolens*
aroma: Sweet, rosy
properties: Antidepressant - Balancing - Uplifting

main uses

mind: Geranium is wonderfully balancing and uplifting for the emotions. It dispels stress and tension and lifts depression.

body:

circulatory
· Poor circulation
· Haemorrhoids
· Varicose veins

reproductive
· PMS
· Menopause

skin
· All skin types
· Balances sebum
· Cellulite
· Eczema

· Burns
· Shingles
· Bleeding
· Chilblains
· Dermatitis
· Head lice
· Insect repellent

urinary
· Infections such as cystitis
· Fluid retention
· Tonic
· Kidney problems

blends well with: Cypress, rose, bergamot, neroli, sandalwood
contraindications: None
price: Medium price range

ginger
'the warmer'

botanical name: *Zingiber officinale*

aroma: Aromatic, hot, spicy, warming

properties: Digestive - Stimulant - Invigorating

main uses

mind: Ginger sharpens the senses and aids the memory. It counteracts coldness, indifference and apathy, boosting confidence and gives us a kick start!

body:

circulatory
· Poor circulation

digestive
· Nausea
· Food poisoning
· Stomach cramps
· Tones and settles the digestion
· Flatulence

· Loss of appetite
· Hangovers
· Indigestion

muscles/joints
· Arthritis
· Rheumatism
· Pain
· Stiffness
· Conditions aggravated by the damp
· Cramps
· Muscle spasms

respiratory
· Clears mucus
· Sinusitis
· Colds and flu
· Bronchitis
· Chills
· Asthma
· Throat problems

blends well with: Lemon, lavender, rosemary, rose, sandalwood

contraindications:
· Use in low dilution for sensitive skin

price: Medium price range

grapefruit
'cleanse and tone'

botanical name: *Citrus paradisi*

aroma: Fresh, citrus, refreshing

properties: Antidepressant - Detoxifying - Uplifting

main uses

mind: Grapefruit has an uplifting effect on the emotions lifting depression and inducing euphoria. It relieves nervous exhaustion, lifts tiredness (e.g. jet lag) and boosts confidence.

body:

digestive
· Detox
· Obesity
· Balances appetite
· Digestive tonic

muscles/joints
· Arthritis
· Gout
· Rheumatism

· Stiffness

reproductive
· PMS

urinary
· Fluid retention
· Toxins

skin
· Oily skin
· Cellulite
· Acne
· Skin tonic

blends well with: Juniper, fennel, neroli, petitgrain, geranium

contraindications:
· Take care with sensitive skin

price: Low price range

jasmine
'confident and sensual'

botanical name: *Jasminum officinale*
aroma: Heady, exotic, floral, sensual
properties: Antidepressant -
Aphrodisiac - Uplifting
main uses
mind: Jasmine is widely used for
nervous problems. It lifts even the
darkest moods and warms the
emotions, inducing optimism,
confidence and euphoria. It releases
inhibitions and is a powerful
aphrodisiac.

body:
reproductive
· Menstrual
 cramps
· Excellent for
 use during
 childbirth
· Frigidity and
 impotence
· Promotes milk
 production

skin
· All types of skin
· Dry
· Sensitive
· Inflamed, red
 skin
· Increases
 elasticity
· Stretchmarks
· Scars

blends well with: Geranium,
mandarin, neroli, sandalwood
contraindications: None
price: High price range. Expensive
but worth it!

juniper berry
'the big cleanse'

botanical name: *Juniperus communis*
aroma: Fresh, woody
properties: Antiseptic - Detoxifying
- Purifying - Tonic
main uses
mind: Juniper clears waste from the
mind just as it does from the body. It
dispels negativity, nervous exhaustion
and revitalises and strengthens
nerves.

body:
digestive
· Over-indulgence
· Detoxification
· Flatulence
· Loss of appetite
· Constipation
· Stomach upsets
· Food poisoning
· Loss of appetite
· Obesity
muscles/joints ·
Arthritis
· Gout
· Rheumatism

· Stiffness
· Pain
skin
· Cellulite
· Oily skin
· Blocked pores
· Haemorrhoids
· Eczema
· Psoriasis
urinary
· Cystitis
· Fluid retention
· Prostate
 problems
· Kidney
 problems

blends well with: Cypress,
fennel, lemon, bergamot, geranium,
frankincense, cedarwood
contraindications:
· Avoid during pregnancy
· Avoid if you have a history of
 kidney disease.
price: Medium to high price range

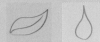

lavender
'the ultimate balance

botanical name: *Lavendula officinalis / augustifolia / vera*

aroma: Sweet, floral, clean

properties: Balancing - Calming - Healing

main uses

mind: Lavender has a remarkable balancing effect on the mind, calming and soothing the emotions. It dispels anger, brings feelings under control and helps us to look at situations from a new perspective. It embodies peace and harmony.

body:

circulatory
· High blood pressure
· Palpitations

digestive
· Nausea
· Flatulence
· Calms the digestive system
· Stomach ulcers
· Indigestion
· Liver problems
· Obesity

muscles/joints
· All muscular aches and pains
· Rheumatism
· Gout

· Arthritis
· Headaches
· Sprains
· Strains
· Muscle spasms

reproductive
· PMS
· Menopause
· Childbirth

respiratory
· Asthma
· Throat infections
· Coughs and colds
· Bronchitis
· Sinusitis
· Flu

skin
· All skin types

· Mature skin
· Stretchmarks
· Sensitive skin
· Eczema
· Psoriasis
· Boils
· Scabies
· Chicken pox
· Athlete's foot
· Burns
· Scars

urinary
· Cystitis
· Fluid retention

blends well with: Bergamot, chamomile, neroli, sandalwood, cedarwood

contraindications: None

price: Medium price range

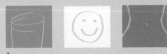

lemon
'clean and refreshing'

botanical name: *Citrus limonum*

aroma: Fresh, sharp, fruity

properties: Detoxifying - Purifying - Tonic

main uses

mind: Lemon clears the mind and dispels lethargy and sluggishness. A refreshing, lively essential oil.

body:

circulatory

· High blood pressure

· Varicose veins

· Hardening of the arteries

· Boosts immune system

· Overall tonic

digestive

· Indigestion

· Stomach ulcers

· Liver/gallbladder problems

· Obesity

· Flatulence

muscles/joints ·

Arthritis

· Gout

· Rheumatism

respiratory

· Coughs

· Colds and flu

· Bronchitis

· Throat problems

· Asthma

· Catarrh

· Sinusitis

· Headaches

skin

· Cuts and wounds

· Oily skin

· Freckles

· Wrinkles

· Stops bleeding

· Acne

· Boils

· Warts

· Cellulite

· Herpes

· Chillblains

· Insect bites

urinary

· Infections

· Thrush

· Fluid retention

blends well with: Cypress, Juniper, frankincense, chamomile, myrrh, neroli

contraindications:

· Do not apply prior to sunbathing

price: Low price range

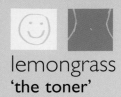

lemongrass
'the toner'

botanical name: *Cymbopogan citratus*

aroma: Astringent, refreshing, sherbet-like

properties: Astringent - Revitalising - Tonic

main uses

mind: Lemongrass refreshes the mind and helps to combat mental fatigue and nervous exhaustion. It spurs you into action!

body:

circulatory
· Poor circulation
· Boosts immune
. system

digestive
· Indigestion
· Loss of appetite
· Colitis
· Flatulence

muscles/joints
· Tones muscles

· Over exercising
· Sprains and strains
· Tired, achy legs

respiratory
· Infections
· Sore throats

skin
· Loose skin, e.g. after dieting
· Enlarged pores

· Excessive sweating
· Athlete's foot
· Oily skin
· Cellulite
· Scabies
· Measles
· Insect repellent

blends well with: Geranium, rosemary, cypress, ginger

contraindications:
· Take care with hypersensitive skin

price: Low price range

mandarin
'the joy of a child'

botanical name: *Citrus reticulata*

aroma: Sweet, floral, delicate, cheery

properties: Balancing - Joyful - Uplifting

main uses

mind: Mandarin banishes depression and negativity, filling us full of love, hope and joy.

body:

digestive
· Tonic for the digestive system
· Obesity
· Stomach cramps
· Loss of appetite
· Hiccups
· Liver/gallbladder problems

reproductive
· Pregnancy (morning sickness and stretchmarks)
· PMS

skin
· Rejuvenation
· Mature skin
· Stretchmarks
· Acne
· Oily skin
· Tonic

blends well with: Lavender, geranium, neroli, lemongrass, rose

contraindications:
· Do not apply prior to sunbathing

price: Low to medium price range

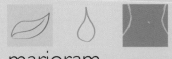

marjoram
'the supreme sedative'

botanical name: *Origanum marjorana*

aroma: Sweet, warming

properties: Calming - Sedative - Warming

main uses

mind: Marjoram clears the mind of stress and anxiety, promoting a deep and restful night's sleep. It is a comforting oil, easing sadness and soothing the broken-hearted.

body:

circulatory
· High blood pressure
· Poor circulation
· Heart tonic

digestive
· Stomach cramps
· Constipation
· Flatulence
· Indigestion
· Nausea

muscles/joints
· Muscle spasms e.g. cramp
· Sprains and strains
· Tired muscles
· Stiffness
· Arthritis
· Rheumatism
· Bruises

reproductive
· Irregular periods
· Painful periods
· Vaginal discharges
· Reduces sexual desire

respiratory
· Loosens mucus
· Colds and flu
· Bronchitis
· Coughs

blends well with: Bergamot, benzoin, lavender, rosemary, frankincense

contraindications:
· Avoid during pregnancy

price: Medium price range

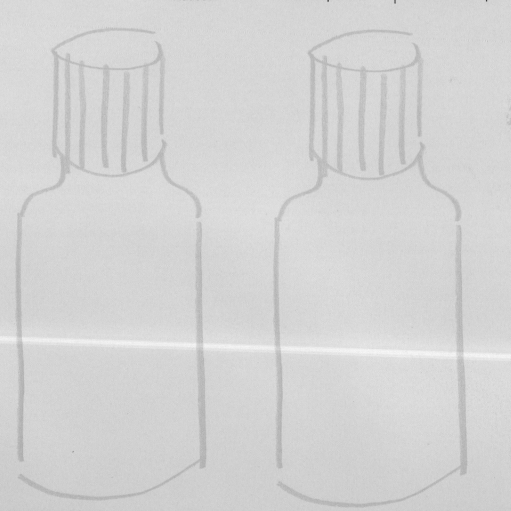

myrrh
'mysterious and healing'

botanical name: *Commiphora myrrha*

aroma: Warm, musty, balsamic, smoky

properties: Anti-catarrhal - Healing - Rejuvenating

main uses

mind: Myrrh banishes apathy and lethargy from the mind and instills strength and courage. It opens up the mind to the mysteries of life.

body:

digestive
· Irritable bowel syndrome (IBS)
· Flatulence
· Diarrhoea

reproductive
· Absence of menstruation
· Tonic for the womb
· Painful menstruation

respiratory
· Colds and flu
· Bronchitis
· Coughs
· Mucus
· Throat problems
· Loss of voice
· Mouth ulcers
· Inflamed gums

skin
· Mature skin
· Cracked/ chapped skin

· Cuts and wounds
· Oily skin
· Wrinkles
· Haemorrhoids
· Athlete's foot
· Eczema
· Dermatitis

blends well with: Frankincense, rose, bergamot, lemon

contraindications:
· Avoid during pregnancy

price: Medium to high price range

neroli
'the ultimate de-stresser'

botanical name: *Citrus aurantium*

aroma: Fresh, floral, haunting

properties: Antidepressant - Aphrodisiac - Calming

main uses

mind: Neroli is one of the most effective oils for nervous problems. It calms highly charged emotional states and instills a feeling of confidence and euphoria. Neroli is excellent for panic attacks and shock.

body:

circulatory
· Palpitations
· High blood pressure
· Heart conditions

digestive
· Muscle spasm
· Colic
· Nervous indigestion

· Diarrhoea
· Butterflies in the stomach

skin
· All skin types
· Dry skin
· Inflamed skin
· Sensitive skin
· Rejuvenating
· Scars
· Thread veins

blends well with: Frankincense, chamomile, citrus oils, geranium, rose

contraindications: None

price: High price range, but worth the investment.

patchouli

'sensuous and rejuvenative'

botanical name: *Pogostemon patchouli*

aroma: Strong, earthy, musty

properties: Antidepressant - Rejuvenating - Soothing

main uses

mind: Patchouli dispels anxiety and stress, instilling peace and calm and clearing away confusion. It combats lethargy and indifference, fills one full of vigour and stimulates sexual desire.

body:

digestive
· Weight reduction
· Irritable bowel syndrome
· Diarrhoea
· Constipation
· Bloatedness

reproductive
· Stimulates libido

skin
· Tissue regeneration
· Mature, aging skin
· Cracked, chapped skin
· Allergies
· Loose skin
· Scars
· Acne
· Dermatitis
· Eczema
· Haemorrhoids
· Athlete's foot
· Dandruff

blends well with: Geranium, neroli, citrus oils

contraindications: None

price: Low to medium price range

peppermint
'the big cooler'

botanical name: *Mentha piperita*

aroma: Cool, piercing, menthol

properties: Cooling - Pain relieving - Stimulating

main uses

mind: Peppermint stimulates the mind, eradicating mental fatigue and aiding concentration and memory. It is a good remedy for shock since it strengthens yet numbs the nerves.

body:

digestive
· All digestive disorders
· Indigestion
· Nausea
· Flatulence
· Heartburn
· Stomach cramps
· Loss of appetite
· Bloating
· Halitosis

muscles/joints
· Headaches (cooling effect)
· All muscular aches and pains
· Neuralgia
· Rheumatism
· Sprains and strains
· Muscle spasms

· Arthritis

reproductive
· Painful menstruation
· Scanty menstruation

respiratory
· Colds and flu
· Sinusitis
· Throat infections
· Bronchitis
· Asthma

skin
· Burns
· Redness and irritation
· Itching
· Acne
· Dermatitis
· Scabies

blends well with: Chamomile, lavender, lemon

contraindications:
· Take care with sensitive skin
· Store away from homeopathic medications
· Avoid when breastfeeding as it could discourage the flow of milk
· Do not use on babies and young children

price: Low to medium price range

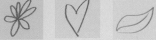

rose
'the scent from heaven'

botanical name: *Rosa centifolia / Rosa damascena*

aroma: Exquisite, heady, intoxicating

properties: Antidepressant - Aphrodisiac - Rejuvenating

main uses

mind: The luxurious and erotically sensuous fragrance of rose makes a woman feel like a woman – confident, positive and sexy. Rose alleviates depression, encouraging feelings of well-being and harmony. It drives out grief and sadness.

body:

circulatory
· Improves circulation
· Cleanses the blood
· Regulates the heart

digestive
· Constipation
· Stomach problems
· Liver disorders

reproductive
· All female disorders
· Cleanses the womb
· Impotence and frigidity
· Menopause
· PMS
· Irregular menstruation
· Painful menstruation

skin
· All skin care
· Mature skin
· Dry skin
· Sensitive skin
· Thread veins
· Capillaries
· Eczema

blends well with: Bergamot, cypress, geranium, mandarin, chamomile

contraindications: None

price: High price range. Rose otto is more expensive than rose absolute.

rosemary
'the restorer'

botanical name: *Rosmarinus officinalis*

aroma: Clean, strong, invigorating

properties: Pain-relieving - Restorative - Stimulating

main uses

mind: Rosemary awakens the brain, clearing the head of mental confusion and promoting clarity. It may help to restore memory loss.

body:

circulatory
· Poor circulation
· Low blood pressure
· Heart tonic
· Palpitations
· High cholesterol

digestive
· Indigestion
· Stomach cramps
· Colitis
· Constipation
· Flatulence
· Over-indulgence in rich food
· Liver/gallbladder problems
· Obesity
· Food poisoning
· Restores appetite

muscles/joints
· Arthritis
· Gout
· Rheumatism
· Muscular aches and pains
· Over-exercised muscles
· Restores muscle tone

reproductive
· Menstrual cramps
· Scanty periods

respiratory
· Colds and flu
· Coughs
· Asthma
· Bronchitis

skin
· Skin toner
· Oily hair
· Dandruff
· Hair loss
· Acne
· Head lice
· Scabies

urinary
· Fluid retention

blends well with: Frankincense, cypress, black pepper, citrus oils

contraindications:
· Avoid during pregnancy
· Do not use extensively on epileptics

price: Low to medium price range

sandalwood
'gently does it'

botanical name: *Santalum album*
aroma: Sweet, woody, warm
properties: Antidepressant - Calming - Soothing
main uses
mind: Sandalwood is renowned for its ability to calm and soothe tension and anxiety, gently soothing away fears and worries. It is excellent for meditation, creating a sense of profound peace.

body:
reproductive
· Aphrodisiac
· Vaginal
  discharges
respiratory
· Asthma
· Bronchitis
· Catarrh
· Coughs (dry)
· Throat
  infections

skin
· All skin types
· Acne
· Oily skin
· Dry skin
· Mature skin
· Cracked and
  chapped skin
· Broken veins
urinary
· Fluid retention
· Infections such
  as cystitis

blends well with: Rose, frankincense, cypress, neroli, geranium
contraindications: None
price: Medium price range

tea tree
'the first aid kit'

botanical name: *Melaleuca alternifolia*
aroma: Sharp, strong, medicinal
properties: Antiseptic - Stimulating
main uses
mind: Tea tree clears the mind, relieves nervous exhaustion and is useful after shock.
body:
circulatory
· Immuno booster
· Glandular fever
· M.E. (post-viral syndrome)
· Varicose veins

reproductive
· Thrush
· Itching
· Vaginal
  discharges
respiratory
· Colds and flu
· Coughs
· Catarrh
· Bronchitis
· Asthma
· Sinusitis
· Throat
  infections

skin
· Cuts and
  wounds
· Acne
· Athlete's foot
· Corns and
  calluses
· Verrucae
· Warts
· Nail infections
· Chicken pox
· Dandruff
· Cold sores
· Shingles

· Rashes
· Psoriasis
· Abscess
· Insect bites
urinary
· Cystitis and other infections
blends well with: Bergamot, juniper, myrrh, sandalwood, thyme
contraindications: None
price: Low to medium price range

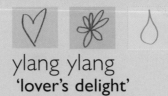

ylang ylang
'lover's delight'

botanical name: *Cananga odorata*

aroma: Sweet, floral, exotic, heavy

properties: Antidepressant - Aphrodisiac - Euphoric

main uses

mind: Ylang ylang is extremely sensuous and provides a very powerful aphrodisiac. It also releases anxiety, tension, anger and fear. Ylang ylang dissipates depression and creates a feeling of confidence and euphoria.

body:

circulatory
· High blood pressure
· Irregular heart beat
· Palpitations

reproductive
· Impotence and frigidity
· Tonic for the uterus

respiratory
· Slows down breathing

skin
· All skin types
· Oily skin
· Dry skin
· Combination skin
· Promotes hair growth

blends well with: Citrus oils, frankincense, rose, jasmine, geranium

contraindications: None

price: Medium price range

chapter three

aroma massage

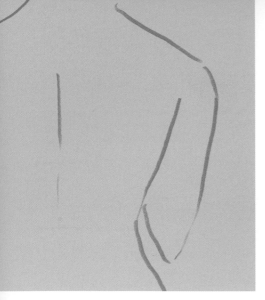

aroma massage

massage is highly therapeutic even without the use of essential oils and is recognised as the oldest form of physical medicine known to man.

The effects of massage are enormous on physical, emotional and spiritual levels, and are an expression of our innate and instinctive ability to comfort and heal. All the systems of the body derive benefit. Massage improves the circulation, bringing fresh nutrients and oxygen to the cells and taking away carbon dioxide and waste products. The lymphatic system is stimulated, enabling the elimination of toxins. The skin improves in texture and tone as dead skin cells are removed, encouraging regeneration. Tense muscles are relaxed as knots and nodules are broken down and joints become much more mobile. Massage encourages deeper breathing and the elimination of mucus and bronchial secretions. Digestion is improved and relief obtained from conditions such as indigestion, constipation and irritable bowel syndrome. Fluid retention is reduced and the function of the kidneys improves. Menstrual problems such as scanty, heavy or painful menstruation are alleviated and the symptoms of the menopause and PMS may be reduced and alleviated. All stress-related conditions such as headaches, insomnia, palpitations and high blood pressure will improve with regular massage. In short, massage is an excellent way to achieve optimum health and well-being.

A massage with aromatherapy oils is even more powerful, as it combines the benefits of therapeutic massage with the healing properties of essential oils.

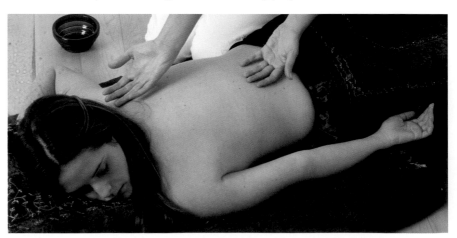

creating a healing environment

1. Choose a peaceful, quiet room with a relaxing ambience.
2. Preheat the room so that the temperature is warm enough for your partner who will be undressed (body temperature drops when lying down).
3. Choose a time when you will be undisturbed - take the telephone off the hook and put a 'do not disturb' notice on the door.
4. Dim the lights or light candles. Harsh, overhead lighting is not conducive to relaxation.
5. Choose some soft, gentle background music for your treatment to encourage both you and your partner to relax.
6. Use an essential oil burner as described on page 33 to set the mood.
7. Enhance the aromatherapy room with a vase of fresh flowers.
8. Make sure that you have everything you will need close at hand – massage oils, creams, essential oils, mixing bowl/bottle, plenty of towels, cushions and pillows.

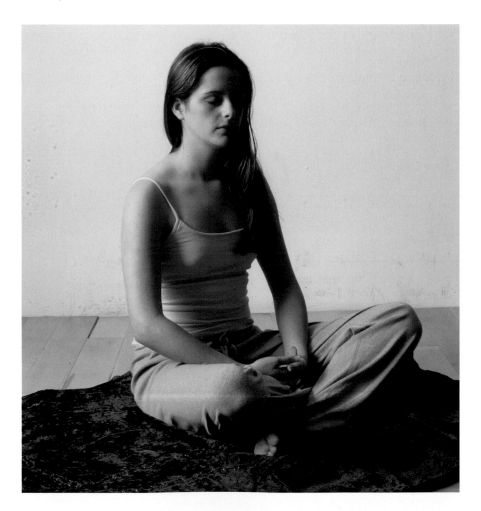

your comfort

It is as relaxing to give an aromatherapy treatment as it is to receive one provided you are comfortable. Wear comfortable, washable clothing – trousers and a tee-shirt are ideal. Do not wear a top with long sleeves since these will get in the way of the aroma massage. Wear flat shoes or go barefoot. Remove all jewellery, especially watches, bracelets and rings with stones which may scratch the receiver. Check that your fingernails are short and will not dig into the receiver; hands and nails should, of course, be scrupulously clean. Finally, make sure that you are relaxed and in a positive state of mind, for negativity and stress may be communicated to the receiver during a treatment.

your partner's comfort

Ask your partner to remove jewellery and to undress down to their underwear. Explain that once he/she is undressed you will be covering them up with lovely warm towels and all they have to do is simply enjoy it!

Use a firm surface like this collapsible massage table.

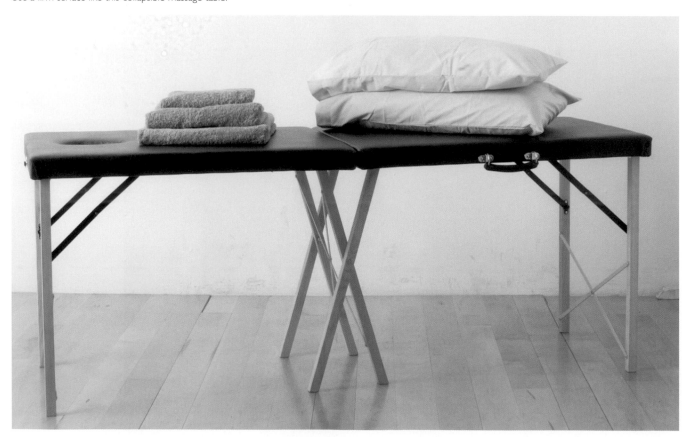

where to massage

A professional aromatherapist will use a purpose-built massage couch to help to prevent back strains. However, do not be disappointed if you do not own one for it is possible to perform a wonderful massage working on the floor. You just need to ensure that you provide adequate padding. A futon, a large piece of foam, a couple of thick blankets/duvet or sleeping bags will all provide the necessary comfort for your partner. Cover the massage surface you have created with a sheet, blanket or towels.

It is possible to use a solid wooden table provided it is sturdy enough and not an awkward height. You will need to cover it with blankets, duvet or sleeping bags to provide comfortable padding.

Massage cannot be carried out on a bed as they are usually far too soft and any pressure that you apply will be absorbed by the mattress.

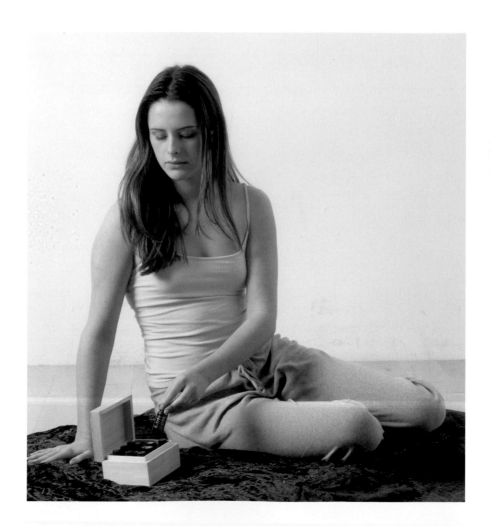

check for contraindications

Although aroma massage is an extremely safe and gentle natural therapy, there are some occasions where it is not advisable or when caution needs to be exercised.

Please observe the following precautions:

1. Never carry out an aroma massage if the person is suffering from a high fever. You could exacerbate the symptoms as the body is already struggling to combat toxins. However, essential oil compresses are excellent.(see page 26).

2. Never treat someone if they are suffering from an infectious illness – you do not want to catch it and pass it on to others.

3. Do not massage a person who is suffering from thrombosis or phlebitis. You could dislodge a blood clot creating a possibility of a heart attack or stroke.

4. Never massage someone with a contagious skin disease such as scabies, ringworm or impetigo.

5. Do not massage over inflamed or swollen areas or you will cause further inflammation. Aromatherapy compresses are excellent for areas of inflammation. A chamomile compress is great for a swollen knee or ankle, for example.

6. Take care over varicose veins.

7. During pregnancy do not massage the abdomen heavily and take particular care during the first three months. Check that the oils you are using are not contraindicated during pregnancy.

8. Beware of recent scar tissue – when the area has healed properly aromatherapy oils are excellent.

9. Do not massage directly over skin eruptions, skin rashes, cuts, wounds, bruises, bites, stings, etc. Essential oils may be used to help heal all of these conditions but it is common sense to avoid these areas as it would cause discomfort and pain.

10. Never massage over broken bones.

11. If someone is suffering from a serious medical condition then seek a doctor's consent.

12. Undiagnosed lumps or bumps should always be checked out by a medically qualified doctor.

13. Do not get the essential oils into either your partner's or your own eyes. If oil does get into an eye then wash it thoroughly with cool water.

14. Make sure that your oils are kept away from children and pets.

15. Take care with particularly sensitive skin – it is a good idea under these circumstances to do a patch test. Mix a drop of your chosen aromatherapy oil with a teaspoon of sweet almond oil and dab it on the crease of the elbow, the inside of the wrist or behind the ear. Leave uncovered and unwashed for 24 hours and then examine the area. If there is no redness, irritation or itching then the oil is safe to use.

16. Avoid exposure to the sun and sunbeds immediately after an aroma massage if you are using citrus oils in your treatment.

17. If your partner suffers from epilepsy check that your chosen oils are not contraindicated.

18. If you are taking homeopathic remedies, do not use peppermint essential oil as it it thought to reduce their effectiveness.

19. Wait a couple of hours after a sauna before enjoying an aroma massage. The pores are open and the body is still eliminating.

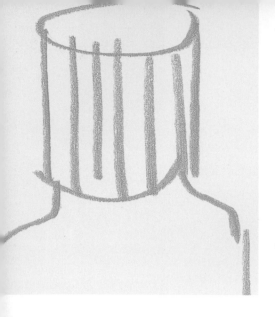

basic aroma massage techniques

the full body aroma massage that is detailed in this book is based on a few classic massage techniques that are simple and easy to learn.

Ask the receiver to lay on his/her front with one pillow under the feet and one under the head. The head may be turned to one side and the arms should be relaxed at the sides. Cover your partner with towels. Keep the prepared and blended aromatherapy oil within easy reach while you practise the techniques. Never pour oil directly onto the body from your bowl or bottle and always warm cold hands by rubbing your hands together vigorously. Simply dip your fingers into your aromatherapy bowl or, if you are using an amber-coloured bottle, pour about half a teaspoon of oil into the palm of one hand. Warm the oil between your palms and then it is ready to apply.

Do not worry if your movements feel a little clumsy or uncoordinated to begin with. The more you practise, the more flowing your movements will become and your confidence will grow.

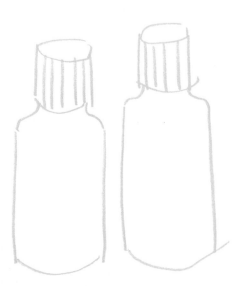

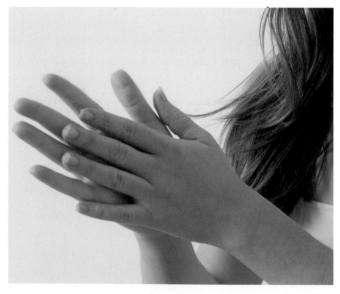

friction

Friction is a marvellous movement for breaking down all those knots and nodules which we all have lurking in our bodies, particularly around the spine and the shoulder blades!

NB When performing friction use only a small amount of oil otherwise your thumbs will slip and slide and you will not be able to feel the knotted muscles.

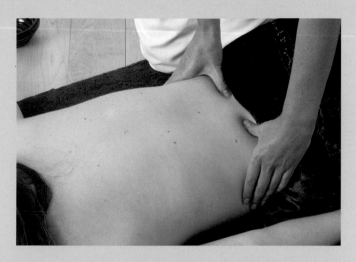

1. Place both hands either side of the spine, with the pads of your thumbs in the dimples at the base of the spine.

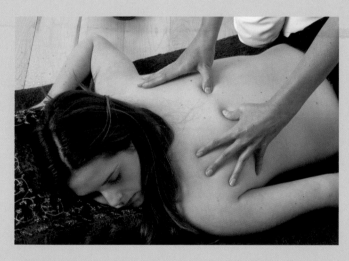

2. Perform small penetrating circular outward movements working up the back towards the base of the neck. As you reach the top glide back to the original position. Expect your thumbs to ache a little until they become accustomed to the pressure. Use your body weight to lean into the movement to achieve a deeper pressure.

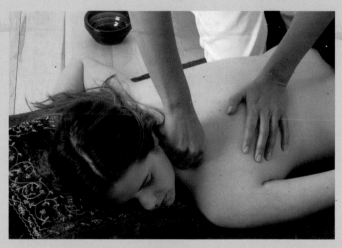

3. Although friction is usually performed with the pads of the thumbs or fingers, the knuckles, the heels of the hand, or even the elbows can also be used. Try circling your knuckles across the tops of the shoulders.

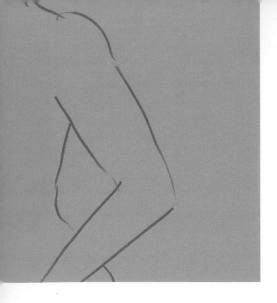

a full body aroma massage

The complete sequence will take you about an hour. However, if your time is limited and you only have15 to 20 minutes to spare, then just choose one part of the body to massage. Favourite areas include the back, face, hands and feet.

Prior to your aroma massage make sure that you have created a relaxing ambience, prepared both yourself and the receiver, and checked for any contraindications (see pages 68).

choosing the right blend

Prepare the aromatherapy blend according to the physical and emotional needs of your partner. Select just one essential oil, or if you wish up to three essential oils, choosing at least one oil for any emotional imbalances. In this way, you will be treating the whole person and not just the symptoms.

Before starting the aroma massage allow the receiver to smell the aromatic formula. Rub a small amount onto the back of your partner's hand. If they like it, it will have a beneficial effect, for we are instinctively drawn to the aroma of the oils which are therapeutic for us at the time. The oils choose you!

Ask the receiver to lie on their front with pillows or cushions placed under the feet and head, and completely cover them with towels. Make sure your hands are warm and you are ready to begin.

I suggest that you mix up 20 ml (4 teaspoons) of carrier oil for a complete sequence – you will probably find you have some oil left over. Remember to use 3 drops of essential oil to 10 ml of carrier oil. This will be sufficient to massage one area of the body. For the complete sequence you will need 6 drops of essential oil to 20 ml of carrier oil.

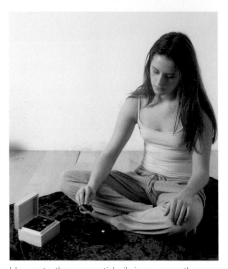

Use up to three essential oils in an aromatherapy massage.

aroma massage on the back of the body

the back

step one – tuning in

Prior to using any oil, position yourself at the side of the receiver and place one hand on the top of the head with the other on the base of the spine.

Gently rest them there for about a minute breathing deeply and gently. This will enable the receiver to become accustomed to your touch and any tension will be released. Notice how you begin to breathe together in unison.

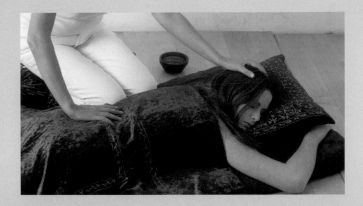

step two – oiling/fan stroking

1. Fold the towel down and apply a small amount of oil (about ½ teaspoon) to the back. Do not be tempted to use too much oil – only apply more if your hands drag the skin. Place both hands, flat down, one either side of the spine, at the bottom of the back with your fingers pointing upwards.

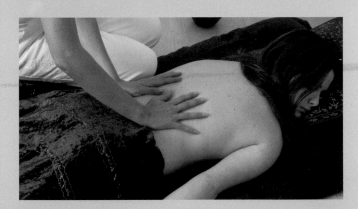

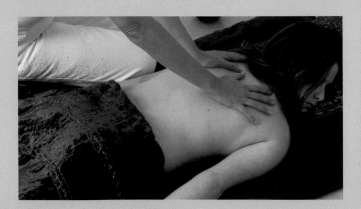

2. Stroke slowly and smoothly up the back, applying an even pressure and leaning into the movement until you reach the neck.

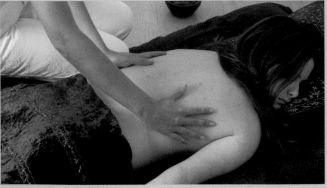

3. As you reach the neck, fan out your hands across the shoulders and then allow them to glide back to the starting point using no pressure whatsoever. Repeat this technique as many times as necessary until your movements feel confident and flowing.

step three – alternate hands fan stroking

1. Place both hands, palms down, one either side of the spine, at the base of the back (same position as in the last technique). Start with your right hand stroking firmly up the back and over the right shoulder and allow it to return effortlessly to the starting position. As your right hand glides gently back, begin stroking up the back with your left hand. One hand strokes up the back the other hand is gliding down the back. Repeat several times, building up a steady rhythm.

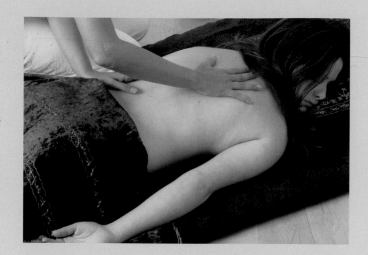

step four – awakening the spinal points

1. Place both hands either side of the spine and place the pads of your thumbs in the dimples at the base of the spine.

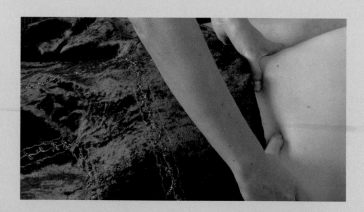

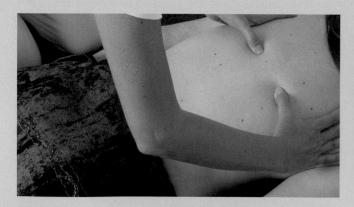

2. Perform small penetrating circular outward movements working up the back towards the base of the neck. As you reach the top glide back to the original position. Expect your thumbs to ache a little until they become accustomed to the pressure. Use your body weight to lean into the movement to achieve a deeper pressure.

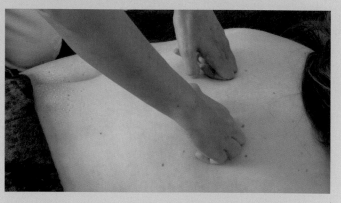

3. Although friction is usually performed with the pads of the thumbs or fingers, the knuckles, heels of the hand or even the elbows can be used, too. If you notice any congested, knotty areas, simply friction over the area with one thumb placed on top of the other. The knuckles may also be used to disperse knots and nodules.

step five – draining away the toxins

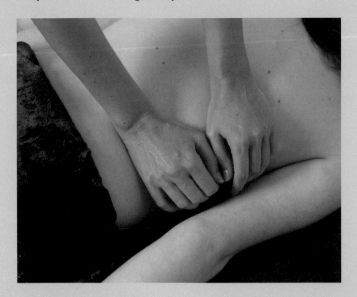

1. Place both hands palms down at the bottom of the back on the side opposite you. Gently push the toxins down the side of the back and flick them away. Work all the way up the back.

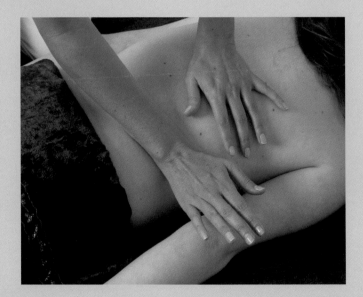

2. Continue draining, but use alternate hands to execute the technique, working up and down the side of the back. One hand should follow closely behind the other to establish a good rhythm. Repeat on the other side.

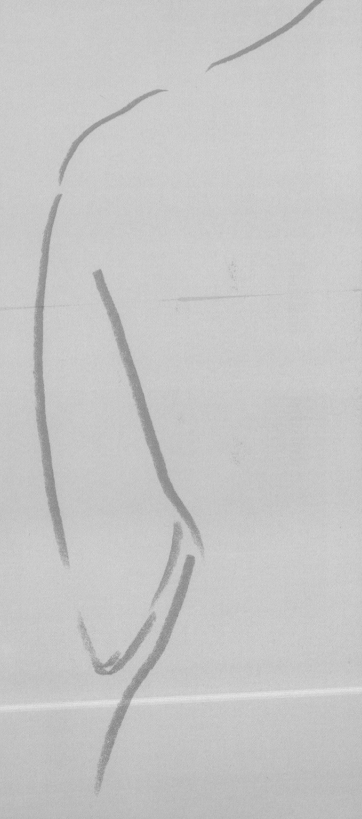

step six – decongesting the lower back

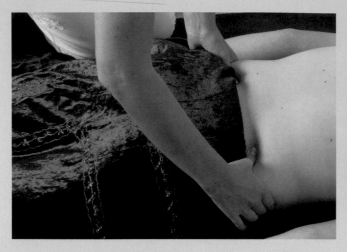

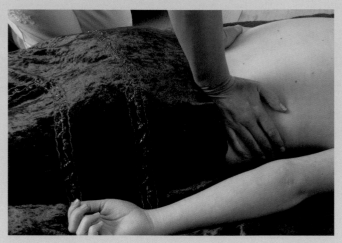

1. Place the pads of your thumbs in the two dimples at the base of the spine. Perform small, deep, outward circular movements across the top of the pelvis. If you encounter any nodules, friction over the area.

2. Place both hands in the middle of the lower back, heels of the hands together with the fingertips facing outwards. Stroke firmly out and over the hips. Glide the hands back with no pressure. Repeat several times to drain away any toxins you have released.

step seven – awakening and decongesting the shoulder blades

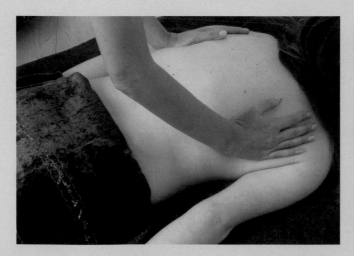

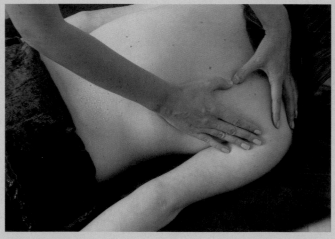

1. Position yourself at your partner's head. Place the palm of your right hand on one shoulder blade and the palm of your left hand on the other one. Make large outward circles with both hands simultaneously.

2. Place the pads of your thumbs on the side of the shoulder blade. Perform deep, circular friction movements all around the rim of each shoulder blade. This will help to release the knots and nodules in the area.

step eight – petrissaging the sides of the back and shoulders

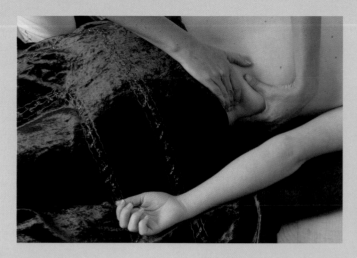

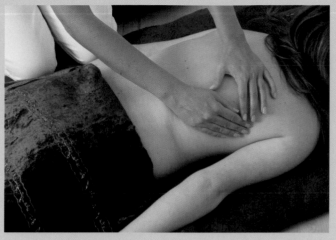

1. Position yourself at the side of the receiver and place both hands flat down on the opposite side of the back on the waist area.

2. Use alternate hands to gently grasp, squeeze and release the flesh using a steady rhythm. Make sure that you are squeezing the flesh and not pinching. Work all the way up the sides of the back, across the shoulders and then work back down again. Repeat on the other side.

step nine – circle stroking

Place both hands on the far side of the back around the shoulder blade, and using the whole of the palms of both hands, begin to circle in a clockwise direction. Begin with the left hand and follow with the right.

Notice that your hands cross over as you perform the circle. Although you will have to lift one hand over the other, make sure that you always keep contact with one hand.

Repeat the circular stroking all the way down the side of the back towards the buttocks and then back up towards the shoulders. Repeat on the other side.

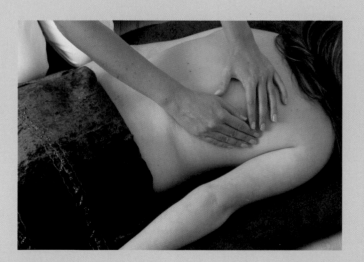

step ten – decongesting the neck

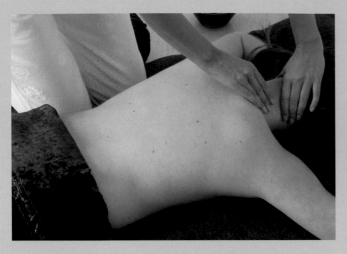

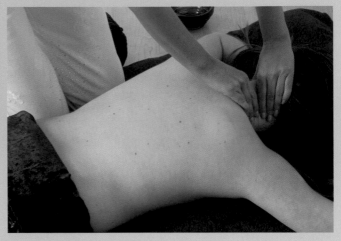

1. Ask the receiver to place their forehead onto their hands to straighten out the neck. A pillow or rolled-up towel under the head is optional.

2. Place both hands flat down, moulding them to the contours of the neck and gently pick up and squeeze the muscles at the back of the neck. Use the whole of your hands, not just your fingers. Both hands may be used at once, or one hand may follow the other.

step eleven – cat stroking

Place the palm of one hand at the base of the receiver's neck. Stroke slowly and smoothly down the back using virtually no pressure.

As one hand reaches the buttocks, gently lift it off and repeat the movement with your other hand. Repeat lots of times – it should feel to the receiver like one continuous movement.

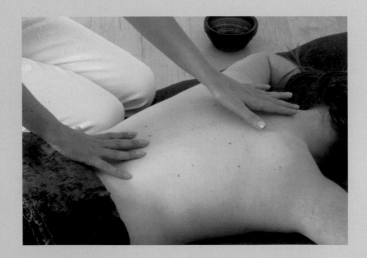

the back of the legs

step one – tuning in

Before drawing back the towel, place the palms gently down one on each leg and hold them there for about 30 seconds or as long as you feel is appropriate.

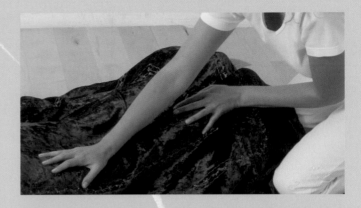

step two – stroking the leg

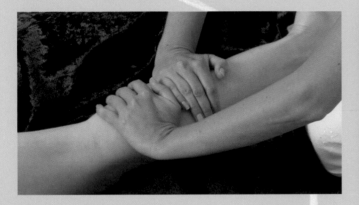

1. Expose one leg and place one hand across the back of the ankle with the fingertips pointing in one direction and your other hand just above with fingertips pointing in the other direction.

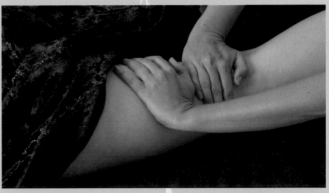

2. Stroke up the leg, moulding your hands to the contours and taking care not to put too much pressure on the delicate area at the back of the knee.

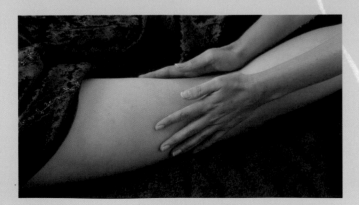

3. As your hands reach the top of the thigh allow them to separate and glide back down the sides of the leg using virtually no pressure.

step three – unblocking the leg

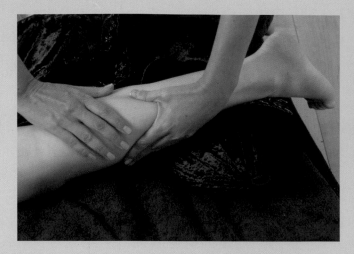

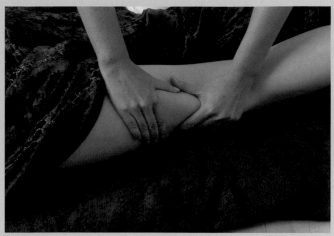

1. Place both hands flat down on the calf muscles. Use alternate hands to pick up, squeeze and release the calf muscles, working smoothly and rhythmically.

2. Continue working up the leg to treat the thigh muscles. Be more vigorous on the outer and middle thigh, and gentle on the inner thigh area.

   These movements will decongest the legs, break down fatty deposits and encourage the elimination of toxins.

step four – fingertip stroking

1. Place the fingertips of one hand at the top of the thigh and stroke gently down with a featherlight touch.

   As one hand reaches the foot, lift it gently off and start stroking with the other hand. With each movement make your touch lighter and lighter. Repeat on the other leg.

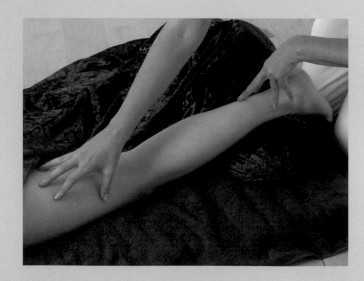

aroma massage of the front of the body

the upper chest, neck and shoulders

step one – tuning in

Position yourself behind the receiver and place both hands gently on the upper chest area. Take a few deep breaths and become aware of the tension and congestion leaving the area.

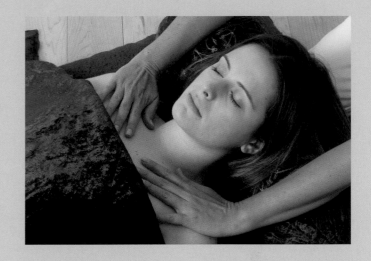

step two – opening up the chest

Apply a small amount of oil to your hands and place them, palms down, just below the collar bones with fingertips pointing towards each other (1). Stroke from the centre of the chest outwards (2) and down towards the lymph glands (3) in the armpits to encourage the elimination of toxins. Allow your hands to glide back to the centre using no pressure.

Repeat several times to ease congestion and relax contracted chest muscles.

1.

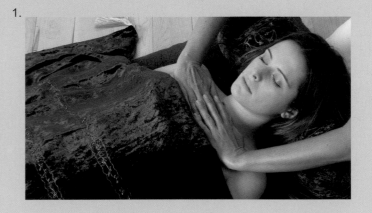

2.

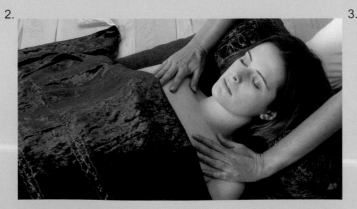

3.

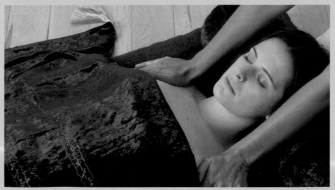

step three – knuckling the chest

Make your hands into loose fists and place them palms down onto the centre of the chest. Perform small circular movements with your knuckles working gently over the chest area. Stroke the area gently again, as in step two.

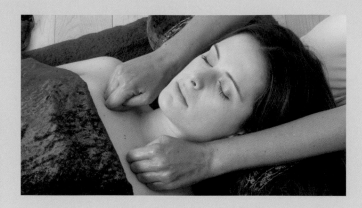

step four – releasing tension from the back of the neck

Place the fleshy pads of your fingers at the base of the skull. Perform small, slow circular movements working down the receiver's neck on either side of the spine. Always avoid pressing on the spine itself.

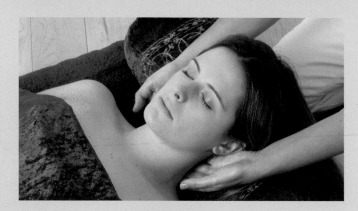

step five – releasing tension from the sides of the neck

1. Ask the receiver to gently turn their head to one side. It is important never to force the neck. Place one hand on the forehead and use your other hand to stroke down the side of the neck.

2. Continue stroking towards and over the shoulder. This movement gives a wonderful stretch to the neck and shoulders. Repeat on the other side of the neck.

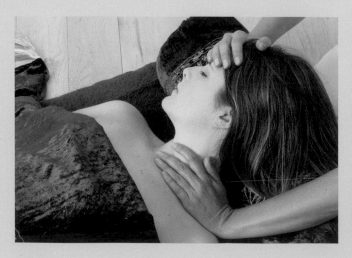

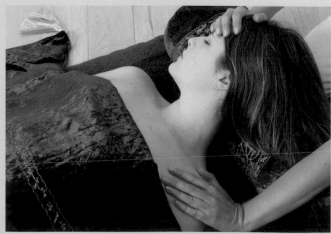

step six – stretching the neck

Ask your partner to move their head back to the middle again so that their neck is straight. Take away the pillow. Cup your hands behind the neck, take the weight of the head in your hands, and very slowly, gently and carefully stretch it towards you. Repeat several times.

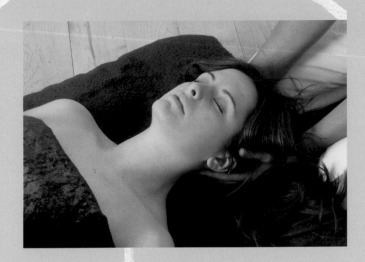

the face and scalp

Aroma massage of the face can take years off your face – it really is a facelift without surgery! Fine lines can be reduced and the face takes on a healthy glow. Headaches can disappear like magic and problems such as sinusitis may be alleviated.

step one – tuning in

Position yourself at the receiver's head and rest the palms of your hands gently on either side of the head. Hold them there for about 30 seconds and feel the anxiety and tension dissipate.

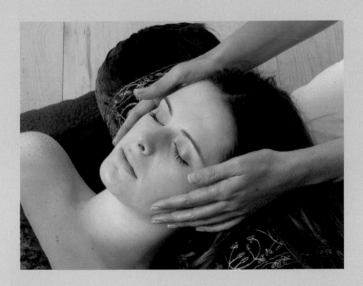

step two – stroking the face

1. Using a minute amount of oil, place the palms of your hands on the forehead, fingers interlocking and stroke outwards.

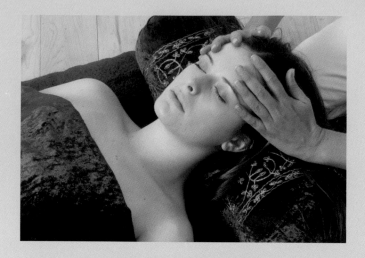

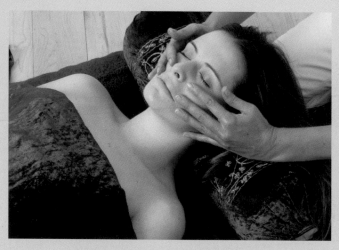

2.With your fingertips stroke outwards across the cheeks.

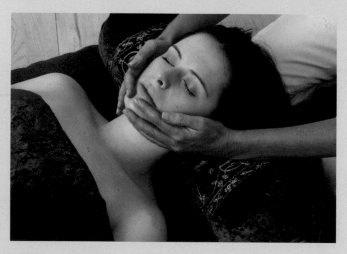

3. Finally, stroke outwards across the chin and continue the movement down the neck.

step three — draining the face

1. Place your thumbs in the centre of the forehead just below the hairline and slide them apart towards the temples. Now repeat this drainage movement on the forehead but this time starting a little lower down. Continue working down the forehead until you reach the eyebrows — this will be approximately four horizontal rows.

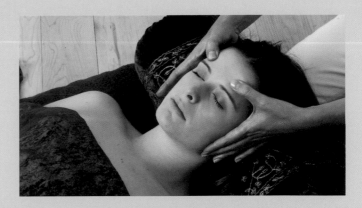

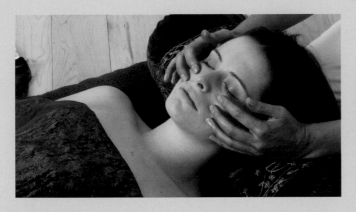

2. Place the pads of your forefingers, middle fingers or both just underneath the inner corners of the eyes. Drain the entire cheek area again working in horizontal strips.

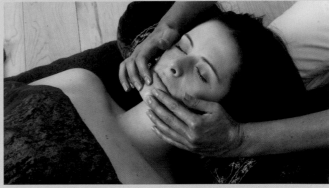

3. To complete the facial decongestion place the thumbs in the centre of the chin and drain outwards in horizontal rows. Then stroke the face again.

step four — decongesting the eyebrows

Use your thumb and index fingers to gently and slowly squeeze the brow bone. Work from the inner to the outer edges.

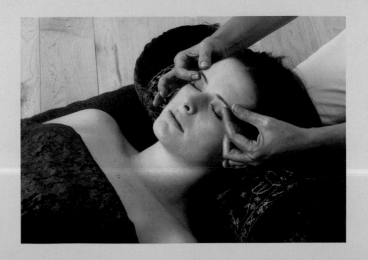

step five – unblocking the nasal passages

Place both thumbs or index fingers at the top of the nose and stroke gently down the sides of the nose several times.

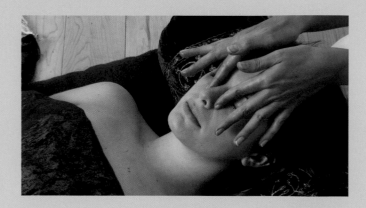

step six – relaxing the jaw

Place your hands in the centre of the jaw, thumbs above and fingers below. Gently pinch the jaw bone, working at regular intervals along the jaw line.

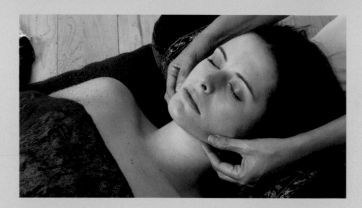

step seven – massaging the ears

Use your thumbs and forefingers to massage all over the ears, and then stretch and release them very gently.

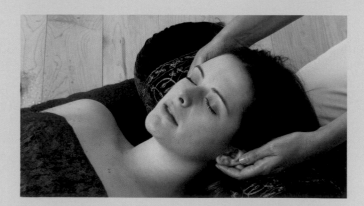

step eight – relieving scalp tension

If the receiver has their hair tied up, then let it down to gain maximum benefit from the scalp massage. Using the fleshy pads of your fingers and thumbs simultaneously, slowly and firmly massage the entire scalp.

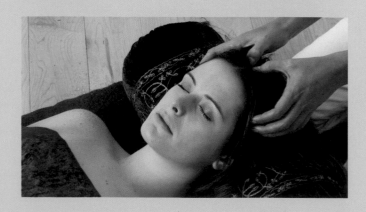

step nine – stroking the hair

Gently run your fingers through the receiver's hair to improve circulation and to release any remaining tension.

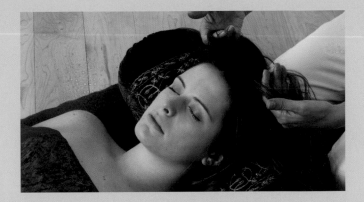

step ten – toning the face and scalp

Use the pads of your fingertips and thumbs to lightly drum all over the scalp, forehead, cheeks and chin.

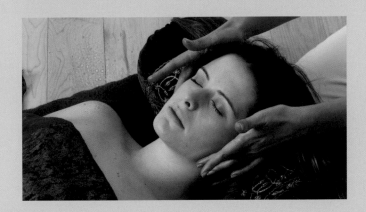

the arms and hands

step one – stroking the arm

Place cupped hands around the receiver's wrist and stroke firmly up the arm towards the lymph glands under the arm. Glide back down the sides with no pressure. Repeat several times.

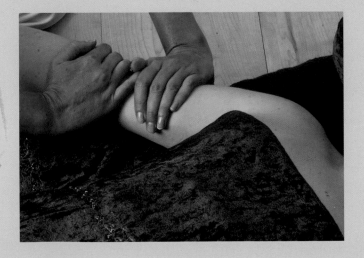

step two – decongesting the arm

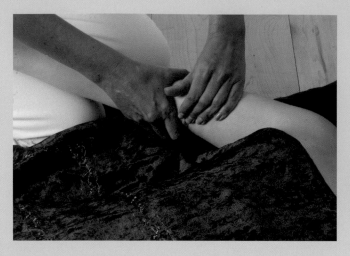

1. Using both hands alternately and rhythmically petrissage the muscles of the upper arms.

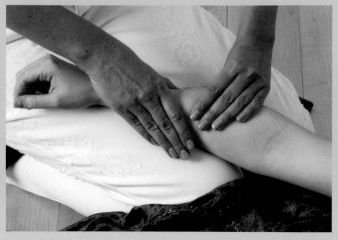

2. Then petrissage the muscles of the forearm.

step three – loosening the hand and wrist with your thumbs

1. Perform small, circular movements all over the back of the hand and the wrist.

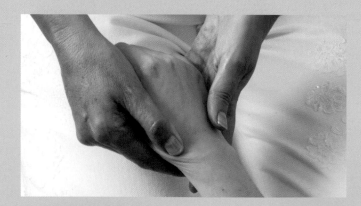

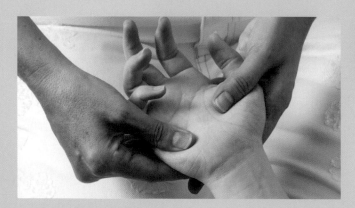

2. Turn the hand over and circle both thumbs all over the palm of the hand and wrist.

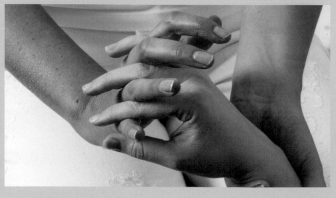

3. Interlock your fingers with your partner and gently and slowly move the wrist clockwise and anticlockwise.

step four – loosening the fingers

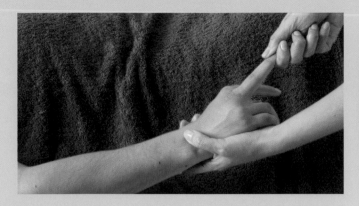 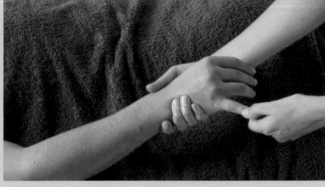

1. Hold your partner's hand palm downwards with one hand and use the thumb and forefinger of your other hand to gently circle up and down each finger and thumb.

2. Rotate the fingers and thumb individually both clockwise and anticlockwise.

step five – fingertip stroking

Using the fingertips of both hands, stroke gently down the arm and hand using the lightest touch.

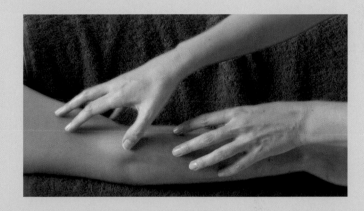

the abdomen

Aroma massage of the abdomen is remarkably effective helping to relieve digestive problems such as constipation, irritable bowel syndrome and indigestion. It is also excellent for abdominal bloating caused by overindulging in too much rich food or by PMS. Abdominal aroma massage also releases tension and encourages deeper breathing.

step one – stroking the arm

Position yourself at the right-hand side of the receiver's abdomen and allow your hands to rest very gently on the navel. Notice how the breathing becomes deeper and more relaxed.

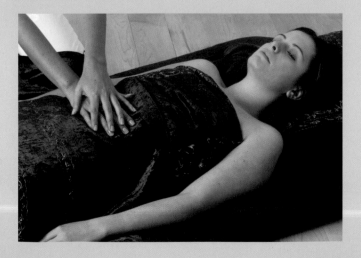

step two – circular stroking

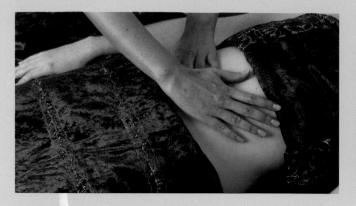 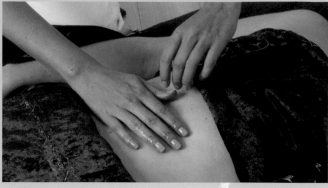

1. Draw back the towel, rub a small amount of the aromatherapy blend between your hands and begin to stroke the abdomen in a clockwise direction using both hands at the same time.

2. As your hands cross over you will need to lift one hand over the other.

step three – pulling up the abdomen

Place both hands under the lower back and gently pull both hands up the sides of the abdomen and then diagonally down towards the bladder. This is a wonderful movement for helping the kidneys and also gives the back a welcome stretch.

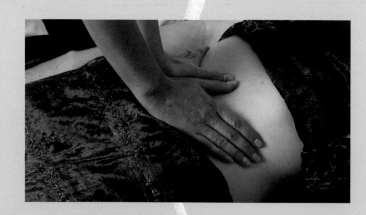

step four – gentle stroking

Use the backs of your hands and fingertips to very gently stroke around the abdomen, scarcely touching the body.

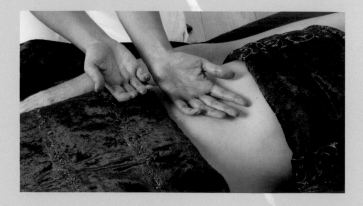

the front of the legs and feet

step one – stroking the leg

Draw back the towel and apply a small amount of oil to your hands. Place cupped hands on top of the ankle and stroke up the entire leg, first with one hand and then with the other, ensuring contact at all times.

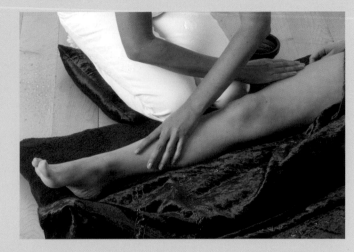

step two – loosening the knee

Use the pads of your thumbs, fingertips or both to work all around the kneecap using small circular pressures.

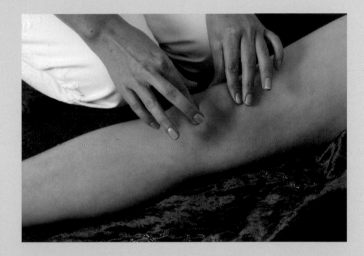

step three – decongesting the thigh

Place both hands palms downwards on the thigh and use alternate hands to pick up, squeeze and release the muscles of the inner, middle and outer thigh. Pay particular attention to the thigh if there is cellulite. Repeat the stroking of the whole leg to eliminate any toxins you have released.

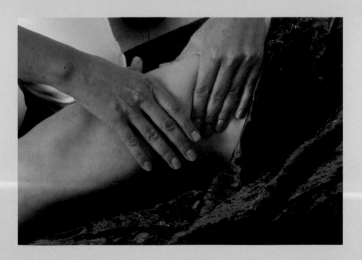

step four – stroking the foot

Apply a minute amount of oil to your hands and stroke firmly up the entire foot using both hands, working from the toes to the ankle. Glide back down gently and repeat the stroking until the foot begins to relax.

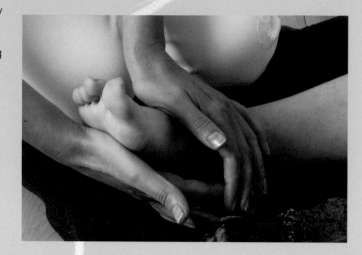

step five – moving the foot

To encourage flexibility of the ankle and to reduce fluid, support the foot with one hand and slowly and gently circle the ankle in both directions.

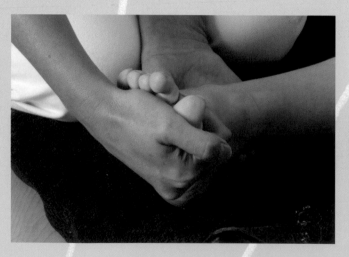

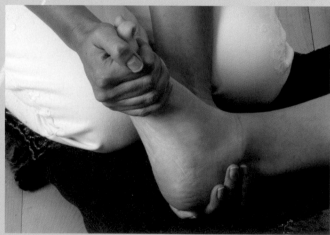

step six – loosening the toes

Support the foot with one hand and use your thumb and index finger to gently squeeze and carefully pull each toe individually towards you to stretch them.

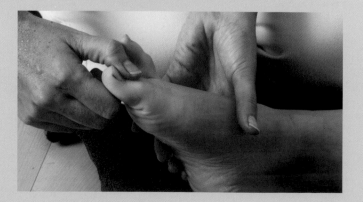

step seven – fingertip stroking

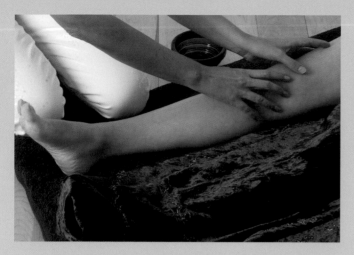

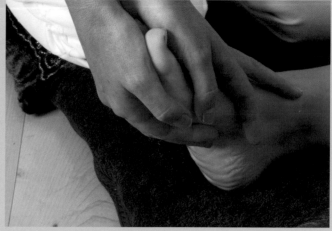

1. Place the fingertips of both hands at the top of the thigh and stroke gently down with a featherlight touch.

2. Repeat several times and gently sandwich the foot between your hands to finish.

Repeat the leg and foot sequence on the other side

completion

To complete your aroma massage use your fingertips to sweep down the whole of the front of the body and off at the toes. Repeat seven times.

Slowly move away from your aroma massage partner and allow him/her to relax and come around gradually.

Always offer your partner a glass of water at the end of the treatment to assist with the detoxification process. Relax after a full aroma massage to derive maximum benefit from the treatment.

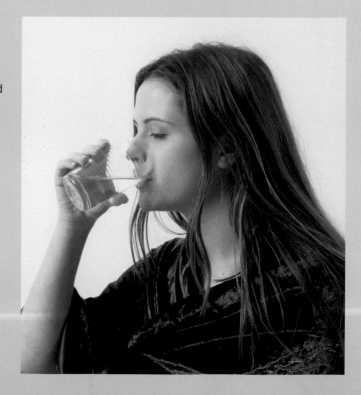

chapter four

aromatherapy for health

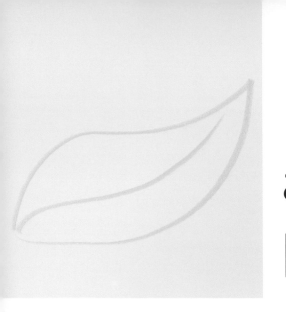

aromatherapy for health

aromatherapy can be used to help alleviate a whole range of physical and emotional health problems, as well as preventing illness from occurring.

In this chapter we will look at the most common ailments occurring in each system of the body and I will recommend appropriate oils for each condition. This chapter will provide you with the tools to prevent and alleviate the majority of everyday health problems simply and effectively. Although these recipes have been tried and tested, if problems persist you must seek medical advice.

There is a brief description of each ailment, along with a list of the recommended oils (which may be used in any of the methods outlined on pages 20–34), an aroma blend and other suggestions for treatment.

aromatherapy for circulatory disorders

anaemia

A common blood disorder characterised by a deficiency of the iron-containing component of the red blood cells. Symptoms include tiredness, sore, smooth red tongue and dry, brittle, spoon-shaped nails.

Suggested aroma massage blend (to 10 ml carrier oil)

Black pepper	1 drop
Chamomile	1 drop
Lemon	1 drop

Further suggestions: a diet high in iron-rich foods such as liver, green leafy vegetables, blackstrap molasses, dried fruits.

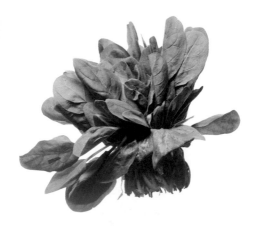

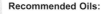

Recommended Oils:

Black pepper,

Chamomile, Lemon,

Angelica, Rose,

Peppermint, Sage,

Thyme.

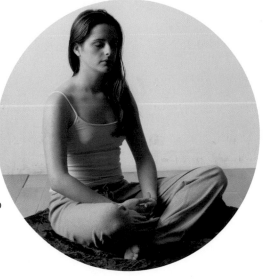

blood pressure (high)

A fairly common disorder with the incidence increasing with age. Symptoms include headaches, dizziness, palpitations, chest pains and visual disturbances.

Suggested aroma massage blend (to 10 ml carrier oil):

Clary sage	1 drop
Frankincense	1 drop
Marjoram	1 drop

Further suggestions: a well-balanced wholefood diet low in salt, sugar, and saturated fats, and high in fruit, vegetables, garlic and dietary fibre. Stress reduction is vital using relaxation techniques, deep breathing, an exercise programme and regular aromatherapy treatments.

Recommended Oils:
Chamomile, Clary sage, Frankincense, Garlic, Lavender, Lemon, Marjoram, Neroli, Rose, Ylang ylang.

blood pressure (low)

Symptoms include dizziness, fainting, tiredness and a tendency to feel the cold.

Suggested aroma massage blend (to 10 ml carrier oil):

Black pepper	1 drop
Peppermint	1 drop
Rosemary	1 drop

Further suggestions: the herbal remedy ginseng may be helpful.

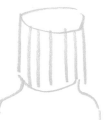

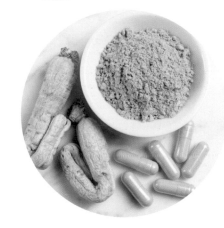

Recommended Oils:
Black pepper, Coriander, Ginger, Hyssop, Peppermint, Rosemary, Sage, Thyme.

circulation (sluggish)

Poor circulation primarily affects the hands and feet and is particularly common in the elderly. It is aggravated by a sedentary lifestyle.

Suggested aroma massage blend (to 10 ml carrier oil):

Black pepper	1 drop
Geranium	1 drop
Ginger	1 drop

Further suggestions: eat plenty of garlic and cayenne pepper, and take lots of exercise.

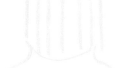

Recommended Oils:
Benzoin, Black pepper, Cypress, Eucalyptus, Garlic, Ginger, Lemon, Lemongrass, Mandarin, Marjoram, Rose, Rosemary, Sage, Thyme.

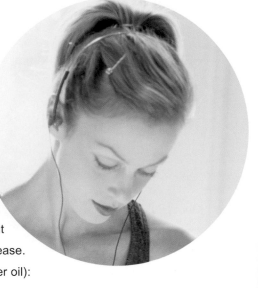

palpitations (anxiety related)

Palpitations, the increased awareness of a strong heart beat, can be due to anxiety and stress. Palpitations should always be checked out by a doctor to eradicate the possibly of heart disease.

Suggested aroma massage blend (to 10 ml carrier oil):

Lavender	1 drop
Sandalwood	1 drop
Ylang ylang	1 drop

Further suggestions: make essential oils and relaxation techniques part of your daily life. Take a B-Complex vitamin supplement and avoid stimulants such as alcohol and caffeine.

Recommended Oils:
Bergamot, Chamomile, Jasmine, Lavender, Marjoram, Melissa, Neroli, Rose, Sandalwood, Ylang ylang.

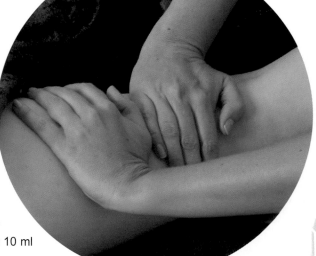

varicose veins

Dilated tortuous veins in the legs affect nearly 50% of middle-aged adults. Prolonged periods of standing, exercise, lifting, obesity, pregnancy, constipation and genetic weakness are all contributing factors.

Suggested aroma massage blend (to 10 ml carrier oil):

Cypress	1 drop
Geranium	1 drop
Lemon	1 drop

NB Massage very gently over an area of veins. Compresses are excellent.

Further suggestions: a high fibre diet, lots of garlic and vitamin C in the form of fresh fruit.

Recommended Oils:
Cypress, Frankincense, Lemon, Geranium, Juniper, Garlic.

aromatherapy for digestive disorders

anorexia nervosa

Most commonly occurs in middle-class teenage girls who become obsessed with their weight. Although painfully thin they perceive themselves as being overweight. In severe cases admission to hospital and tube-feeding is necessary.

Suggested aroma massage blend (to 10 ml carrier oil):

Bergamot	1 drop
Fennel	1 drop
Rose	1 drop

Further suggestions: eat small but frequent meals of nutrient-rich food. Vitamin and mineral supplements (especially zinc) are essential. Referral to a counsellor to get to the cause of the problem.

Recommended Oils:

Bergamot, Fennel,

Black pepper, Lime,

Neroli, Mandarin,

Coriander,

Cardamon.

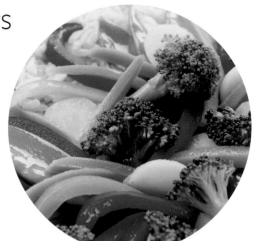

constipation

Difficult or infrequent passing of motions with hard dry stools.

Suggested aroma massage blend (to 10 ml carrier oil):

Black pepper	1 drop
Marjoram	1 drop
Rose	1 drop

Use palmarosa if rose is too expensive.

Further suggestions: eat a healthy, high-fibre diet and drink eight glasses of water daily. Take regular exercise.

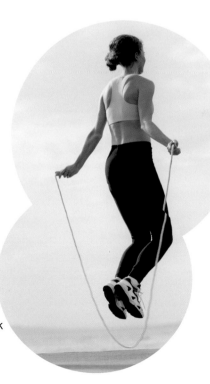

Recommended Oils:

Black pepper,

Cardamon, Fennel,

Ginger, Juniper,

Lemon, Lemongrass,

Marjoram, Palmarosa,

Rose, Rosemary.

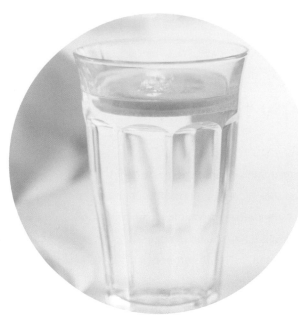

diarrhoea

Too frequent passing of motions. It may be brought on by stress, food poisoning, an infection or an allergy to certain foods.

Suggested aroma massage blend (to 10 ml carrier oil):

Chamomile	1 drop
Ginger	1 drop
Neroli	1 drop

Use petitgrain if neroli is too expensive.

Further suggestions: drink plenty of water, and if it persists see a medically qualified doctor.

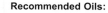

Recommended Oils:

Chamomile, Geranium, Ginger, Lavender, Mandarin, Neroli, Peppermint, Sandalwood.

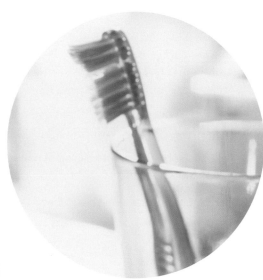

halitosis

Otherwise known as bad breath, halitosis may be caused by eating very spicy foods, poor dental hygiene or by certain digestive disorders.

Suggested aroma massage blend (use a mouthwash – see page 28):

Peppermint	1 drop
Lemon	1 drop

Further suggestions: use the mouthwash daily after brushing the teeth. Chew fennel seeds to sweeten the breath.

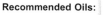

Recommended Oils:

Bergamot, Cardamon, Fennel, Lemon, Parsley, Peppermint, Sage, Spearmint.

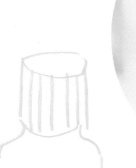

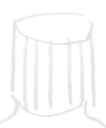

indigestion / heartburn

A burning sensation behind the breastbone caused by over-indulgence, eating too quickly, stress or a food allergy.

Suggested aroma massage blend (to 10 ml carrier oil):

Lemon	1 drop
Ginger	1 drop
Fennel	1 drop

Further suggestions: eat slowly, chew thoroughly and avoid too many rich foods. Do not eat too late at night and avoid stress and tension.

Recommended Oils:

Basil, Bergamot, Cardamon, Chamomile, Coriander, Fennel, Ginger, Grapefruit, Lemon, Lemongrass, Lime, Marjoram, Mandarin, Neroli, Peppermint, Rosemary, Spearmint.

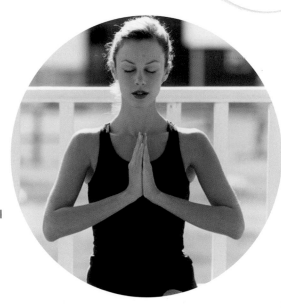

irritable bowel syndrome

Alternating bouts of diarrhoea and constipation, bloating of the abdomen, cramping and flatulence are all symptoms of irritable bowel syndrome. It is related to stress and diet.

Suggested aroma massage blend (to 10 ml carrier oil):

Chamomile	1 drop
Lavender	1 drop
Peppermint	1 drop

Further suggestions: use relaxation techniques such as deep breathing and yoga, and seek regular aromatherapy treatments. Seek the advice of a practitioner who carries out allergy testing.

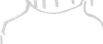

Recommended Oils:

Basil, Chamomile, Geranium, Lavender, Lemongrass, Marjoram, Melissa, Peppermint.

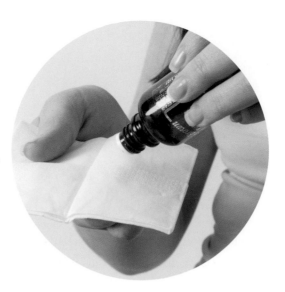

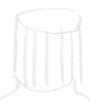

nausea

The sensation of wanting to vomit. This may be
due to gastric upset, stress, mild food poisoning,
pregnancy or may be induced by travel.
Suggested aroma massage blend (to 10 ml
carrier oil):

Chamomile   1 drop
Ginger   1 drop
Peppermint   1 drop

Further suggestions: if you suffer from travel sickness, put a few drops of any of
the above oils onto a handkerchief, tissue or a cotton ball.

Recommended Oils:

Basil, Black pepper,
Cardamon,
Chamomile, Fennel,
Ginger, Lavender,
Mandarin,
Peppermint,
Spearmint.

obesity

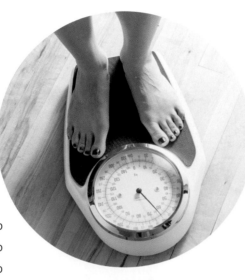

Obesity is a major problem and
is defined as a condition in
which an individual weighs
20% or more above the ideal
weight for their height.
Suggested aroma massage
blend (to 10 ml carrier oil):

Fennel   1 drop
Geranium   1 drop
Lemon   1 drop

Further suggestions: most obesity is caused by overeating and it is essential to
combine a healthy diet with an exercise programme.

Recommended Oils:

Black pepper,
Cardamon, Fennel,
Geranium, Ginger,
Grapefruit, Juniper,
Lemon, Peppermint,
Spearmint.

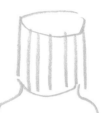

ulcers (stomach)

Ulceration of the lining of the stomach induced by poor diet
and stress.
Suggested aroma massage blend (to 10 ml carrier oil).

Chamomile   1 drop
Lemon   1 drop
Marjoram   1 drop

Further suggestions: reduce stress and avoid acid-producing products such as
coffee, tea, cola and tobacco. Increase fibre in the diet and drink peppermint,
ginger or chamomile tea.

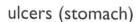

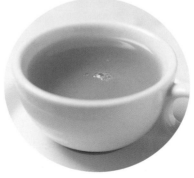

Recommended Oils:

Chamomile,
Geranium, Ginger,
Lavender, Lemon,
Marjoram, Neroli,
Rose.

aromatherapy for the nervous system

anxiety

A general feeling of apprehension caused by stress. Symptoms include palpitations, increased sweating, negative thinking, recurring thoughts, insomnia and irritability.

Suggested aroma massage blend (to 10 ml carrier oil):

Bergamot	1 drop
Frankincense	1 drop
Neroli	1 drop

Use petitgrain if neroli is too expensive.

Further suggestions: learn relaxation techniques such as deep breathing and yoga. Make essential oils part of your daily life – use aromatic baths, inhalations every day and aroma massage at least once a week. Avoid stimulants such as alcohol and caffeine and take a B-complex vitamin supplement.

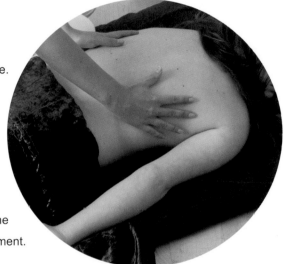

Recommended Oils:

Basil, Bergamot, Chamomile, Clary sage, Cypress, Frankincense, Geranium, Jasmine, Juniper, Lavender, Marjoram, Neroli, Rose, Sandalwood, Vetivert, Ylang ylang.

depression

Symptoms include lack of energy, lethargy, feeling low, sleep problems, loss of interest in life, difficulty in concentrating and feelings of hopelessness and despair.

Suggested aroma massage blend (to 10 ml carrier oil):

Bergamot	1 drop
Geranium	1 drop
Jasmine	1 drop

Use ylang ylang if jasmine is too expensive.

Further suggestions: chronic depression needs professional help such as cognitive behaviour therapy and possibly even antidepressants. Mild depression will respond to regular use of aromatherapy and a good quality vitamin and mineral supplement.

Recommended Oils:

Basil, Bergamot, Cedarwood, Chamomile, Clary sage, Frankincense, Geranium, Lavender, Jasmine, Neroli, Rose, Sandalwood, Ylang ylang and the citrus oils.

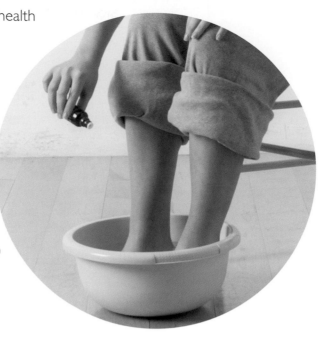

headache

Often caused by nervous or muscular
tension, ranging in intensity from mild
to severe.

Suggested aroma massage blend (to 10
ml carrier oil):

Chamomile	1 drop
Lavender	1 drop
Peppermint	1 drop

Further suggestions: a cold footbath with four drops lavender and two drops
peppermint is an excellent remedy for headaches, as are cool compresses of
lavender on the head and neck.

Try to avoid stress or use relaxation techniques to cope with it.

Recommended Oils:

Chamomile, Clary

Sage, Lavender,

Majoram, Peppermint,

Spearmint.

insomnia

Characterised by difficulty in going to sleep, poor-quality or disturbed sleep,
insomnia is a very common problem. Sufferers will feel fatigued and irritable.

Suggested aroma massage blend (to 10 ml carrier oil):

Lavender	1 drop
Marjoram	1 drop
Neroli	1 drop

Use petitgrain if neroli is too expensive.

Further suggestions: develop relaxation
techniques and do not eat heavy meals, drink
coffee or exercise late at night. Sprinkle a few
drops of lavender on your pillow.

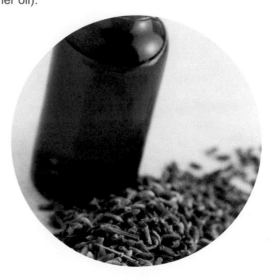

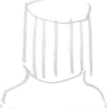

Recommended Oils:

Chamomile, Clary

Sage, Lavender,

Majoram, Neroli,

Petitgrain, Rose,

Sadalwood,

Ylang-ylang.

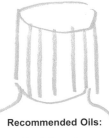

mental fatigue / nervous exhaustion

A feeling of being 'burnt out' caused by overworking or excessive stress.

Suggested aroma massage blend (to 10 ml carrier oil):

Basil	1 drop
Lime	1 drop
Rosemary	1 drop

Further suggestions: use relaxation techniques and try aromatherapy inhalation from a burner or a tissue three times a day. Take time to exercise, develop a regular sleep pattern and have more fun!

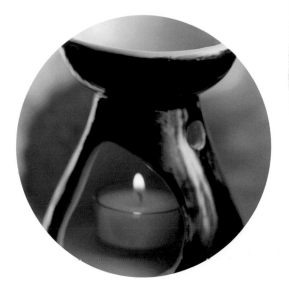

Recommended Oils:

Basil, Benzoin, Eucalyptus, Grapefruit, Juniper, Lavender, Lemon, Lemongrass, Lime, Mandarin, Peppermint, Pine, Rosemary.

migraine

An extremely painful, often one-sided headache accompanied by nausea and visual disturbances. It may be triggered by stress, muscular tension, diet or hormone imbalance.

Suggested aroma massage blend (to 10 ml carrier oil):

Lavender	1 drop
Marjoram	1 drop
Peppermint	1 drop

Further suggestions: try to reduce stress, seek out a practitioner who carries out allergy testing and if symptoms do not improve with aromatherapy massage, osteopathy may be necessary.

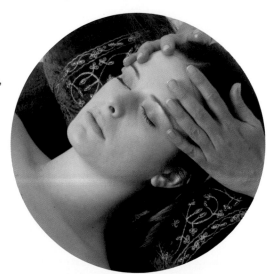

Recommended Oils:

Chamomile, Geranium, Lavender, Marjoram, Peppermint, Spearmint.

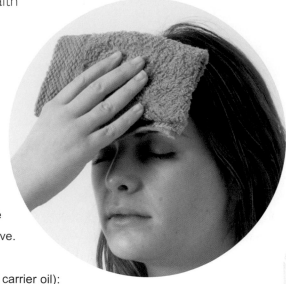

neuralgia

An intense pain along the course of a nerve
caused by irritation or compression of a nerve.

Suggested aroma massage blend (to 10 ml carrier oil):

Chamomile   1 drop

Geranium   1 drop

Peppermint   1 drop

Further suggestions: consult a cranial osteopath and use relaxation techniques.
Compresses should be applied several times daily to the affected area.

Recommended Oils:

Basil, Black pepper,

Chamomile,

Eucalyptus,

Geranium, Lavender,

Marjoram,

Peppermint,

Spearmint, Yarrow.

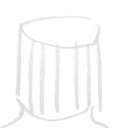

stress

A condition arising when
excessive demands are
made on an individual's
physical and mental energy.
Suggested aroma massage blend
(to 10 ml carrier oil):

Bergamot   1 drop

Geranium   1 drop

Neroli   1 drop

Use petitgrain if neroli is too expensive.

Further suggestions: take a B-Complex vitamin supplement, eat a healthy diet
and use relaxation techniques such as deep breathing. Try not to take on too
much and make time for a regular aromatherapy treatment.

Recommended Oils:

Basil, Bergamot, Clary

sage, Cypress,

Frankincense,

Geranium, Jasmine,

Lavender, Mandarin,

Marjoram, Neroli,

Patchouli, Petitgrain,

Rose, Sandalwood,

Ylang Ylang.

aromatherapy for muscular and joint disorders

arthritis

There are many forms of arthritis. It is a common disorder occurring in almost everyone over the age of 60. It can be caused by wear and tear or overuse and is aggravated by obesity. Symptoms include pain, stiffness, restriction of movement and possibly swelling.

Suggested aroma massage blend (to 10 ml carrier oil):

Black pepper	1 drop
Ginger	1 drop
Juniper	1 drop

Further suggestions: compresses with any of the above oils are excellent for arthritic conditions (see page 24). Daily aromatherapy baths, footbaths or hand baths are recommended. A good diet is vital.

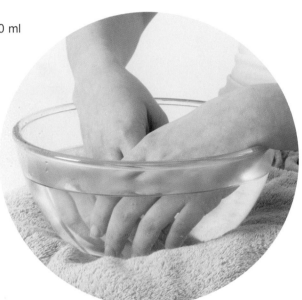

Recommended Oils:

Angelica seed, Benzoin, Black pepper, Cajeput, Chamomile, Eucalyptus, Ginger, Juniper, Lavender, Lemon, Marjoram, Rosemary, Sage, Thyme.

cramp

Spasmodic gripping pain in the muscles that can be mild or severe. Causes include over-exercise, poor circulation, pregnancy, lack of calcium and muscular tension.

Suggested aroma massage blend (to 10 ml carrier oil):

Lavender	1 drop
Marjoram	1 drop
Rosemary	1 drop

Further suggestions: compresses are excellent for immediate relief, as is massage of the legs prior to bedtime.

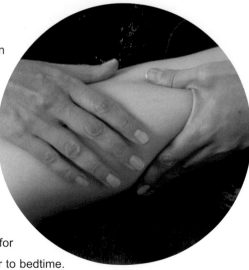

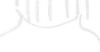

Recommended Oils:

Basil, Black pepper, Cajeput, Chamomile, Cypress, Eucalyptus, Grapefruit, Juniper, Lavender, Marjoram, Peppermint, Rosemary.

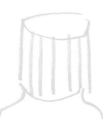

gout

An intensely painful condition causing inflammation commonly affecting the big toe. It is common in men over the age of 40 who over-indulge in wine and food!
Suggested aroma massage blend (to 10 ml carrier oil):

Cajeput 1 drop

Lemon   1 drop

Rosemary   1 drop

Further suggestions: regular aroma massage will help to detox. Diet and lifestyle must be changed if gout is to be prevented.

Recommended Oils:

Angelica seed, Coriander, Carrot seed, Chamomile, Juniper, Lemon, Rosemary.

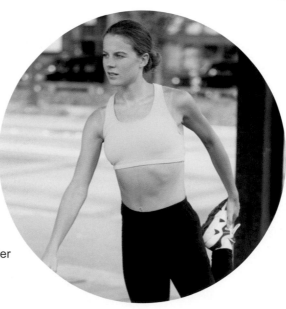

muscular aches and pain

A common problem experienced by all of us and mainly caused by over-exertion. It may also be due to stress and tension, poor posture or arthritis or rheumatism.

Suggested aroma massage blend (to 10 ml carrier oil)

Black pepper   1 drop
Frankincense   1 drop
Rosemary   1 drop

Further suggestions: for acute sharp pain, try cold compresses and for dull muscular aches and pains use hot compresses (see page 26). Avoid prolonged sitting or standing, take frequent breaks to walk and stretch, lift carefully and exercise regularly. (But do not overdo it!)

Recommended Oils:

Angelica seed, Basil, Benzoin, Black pepper, Chamomile, Eucalyptus, Frankincense, Ginger, Juniper, Lavender, Marjoram, Peppermint, Rosemary, Sage, Thyme.

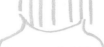

sprains, strains and swollen joints

Swelling and pain are the main symptoms, usually caused by over-used, stretched or wrenched muscles and joints.

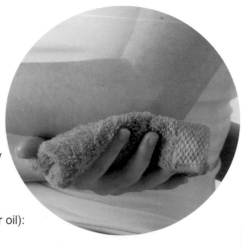

Suggested aroma massage blend (to 10 ml carrier oil):

Chamomile	1 drop
Cypress	1 drop
Ginger	1 drop

Further suggestions: cold compresses are excellent for bringing down swelling on a sprained knee or ankle, for example. (see page 26) The affected part must be rested and elevated.

Recommended Oils:

Black pepper, Chamomile, Cypress, Eucalyptus, Geranium, Ginger, Juniper, Lavender, Marjoram, Peppermint, Rosemary, Sage, Yarrow.

stiffness

Often the result of unaccustomed exercise due to a build-up of waste products.

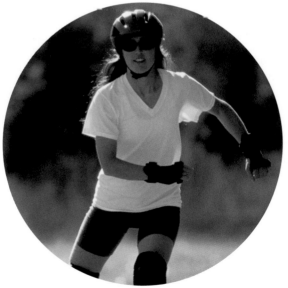

Suggested aroma massage blend (to 10 ml carrier oil):

Ginger	1 drop
Lemongrass	1 drop
Rosemary	1 drop

Further suggestions: always prepare the muscles for exercise and take regular exercise rather than just once a month.

Recommended Oils:

Black pepper, Chamomile, Eucalyptus, Ginger, Juniper, Lavender, Lemongrass, Marjoram, Rosemary.

aromatherapy for reproductive disorders

infertility

The inability to conceive is caused by a wide variety of problems.

Suggested aroma massage blend (to 10 ml carrier oil):

Geranium	1 drop
Jasmine	1 drop
Rose	1 drop

Further suggestions: supplements of zinc have been found to be useful. Try to relax and use essential oils to stimulate your libido.

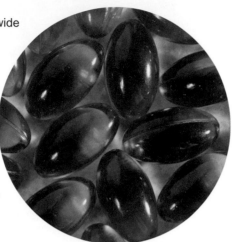

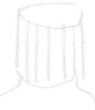

Recommended Oils:

Carrot seed, Clary sage, Geranium, Jasmine, Melissa, Neroli, Rose.

menopause

The menopause usually occurs between the ages of 45–55. The most commonly experienced symptoms include hot flushes, night sweats, scanty or heavy bleeding, irritability, weight gain and depression.

Suggested aroma massage blend (to 10 ml carrier oil):

Cypress	1 drop
Frankincense	1 drop
Rose	1 drop

Use geranium if rose is too expensive.

Further suggestions: the menopause is a normal stage of a woman's development – not an illness – and essential oils can really help! A spray (see page 32) with peppermint is excellent for hot flushes. Take daily baths and have regular aroma massage. Eat calcium-rich foods such as sardines, nuts and dairy products, and take regular exercise.

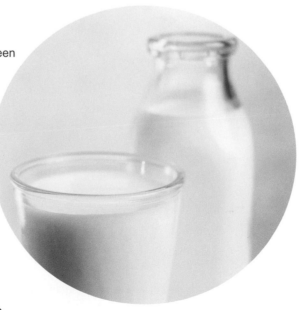

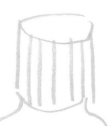

Recommended Oils:

Bergamot, Chamomile, Clary sage, Cypress, Fennel, Frankincense, Geranium, Jasmine, Juniper, Lavender, Melissa, Neroli, Rose, Sandalwood, Ylang ylang.

menstruation

heavy menstruation (menorrhagia)

Profuse bleeding often with clotting.

Suggested aroma massage blend (to 10 ml carrier oil):

Cypress 1 drop

Lemon   1 drop

Rose   1 drop

Use geranium if rose is too expensive.

Further suggestions: Sitz baths are excellent
(see page 25). Beware of anaemia and do check
it out with a medically qualified doctor.

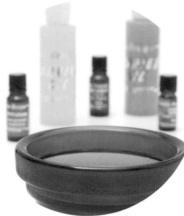

Recommended Oils:

Chamomile, Cypress,

Geranium, Lemon,

Rose.

loss of periods (amenorrhoea / scanty periods)

Loss of periods may be caused by excessive dieting, prolonged stress, strenuous
physical training or coming off the contraceptive pill.

Suggested aroma massage blend (to 10 ml carrier oil):

Cypress   1 drop

Fennel   1 drop

Juniper   1 drop

Further suggestions: eat a healthy diet and use essential oils regularly.

Recommended Oils:

Basil, Clary sage,

Fennel, Juniper,

Marjoram, Myrrh,

Parsley, Rose,

Rosemary, Sage.

painful periods (dysmenorrhoea)

Caused by cramping of the uterine muscles, the pain varies
from a mild ache to a severe incapacitating pain.

Suggested aroma massage blend (to 10 ml carrier oil):

Clary sage   1 drop

Marjoram   1 drop

Peppermint   1 drop

Further suggestions: aroma massage of the
abdomen, sitz baths and compresses are all
excellent. A healthy diet is vital.

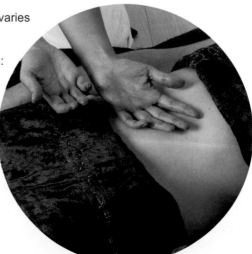

Recommended Oils:

Chamomile, Cajeput,

Clary sage, Cypress,

Jasmine, Juniper,

Lavender, Marjoram,

Melissa, Peppermint,

Rose, Rosemary.

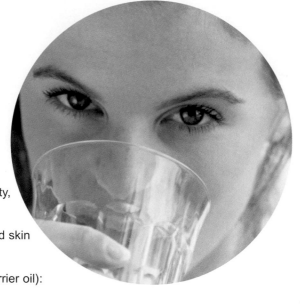

PMS
(pre-menstrual syndrome)

A wide range of symptoms affecting women in the second half of the menstrual cycle. Irritability, mood swings, bloating, breast tenderness, headaches, cravings, lack of concentration, and skin problems are all symptoms.

Suggested aroma massage blend (to 10 ml carrier oil):

Clary sage	1 drop
Cypress	1 drop
Rose	1 drop

Use geranium if rose is too expensive.

Further suggestions: reduce stress with regular use of essential oils, and exercise regularly. Adjust your diet and avoid refined sugar and drinks containing caffeine. Drink three glasses of water daily.

Recommended Oils:

Chamomile, Citrus Oils, Clary sage, Cypress, Frankincense, Geranium, Jasmine, Juniper, Lavender, Marjoram, Neroli, Rose, Sandalwood, Ylang ylang.

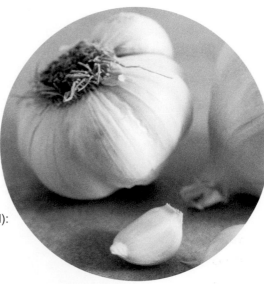

vaginal discharges
(including thrush)

Vaginal discharges are usually white or yellow and may be accompanied by itching and an unpleasant odour.

Suggested aroma massage blend (to 10 ml carrier oil):

Bergamot	1 drop
Lavender	1 drop
Tea tree	1 drop

Further suggestions: take sitz baths (see page 25) several times daily. Eat a healthy diet and incorporate garlic capsule supplements.

Recommended Oils:

Bergamot, Chamomile, Eucalyptus, Frankincense, Juniper, Lavender, Lemon, Myrrh, Sandalwood, Tea tree.

aromatherapy for respiratory disorders

asthma

There is often a family history of asthma and it is usually triggered by an allergy to tree pollen, grass, animal fur, moulds, fungi, dust, chemicals or certain foods. Exercise and stress may also induce an attack.

Suggested aroma massage blend (to 10 ml carrier oil):

Frankincense	1 drop
Lavender	1 drop
Myrrh	1 drop

Further suggestions: adjust your diet and lifestyle, and use aromatherapy extensively to support orthodox medication. Avoid stress and take up breathing exercises and yoga.

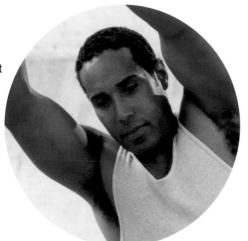

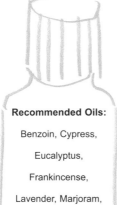

Recommended Oils:

Benzoin, Cypress, Eucalyptus, Frankincense, Lavender, Marjoram, Myrrh, Neroli, Patchouli, Peppermint, Pine, Rosemary.

colds/coughs/flu

These conditions are often accompanied by nasal and bronchial congestion, fever, headache and fatigue.

Suggested aroma massage blend (to 10 ml carrier oil):

Cajeput	1 drop
Cypress	1 drop
Lemon	1 drop

Further suggestions: aromatherapy steam inhalations and chest and back rubs are excellent for colds, coughs and flu. Drink lots of water, honey and lemon drinks and try to rest.

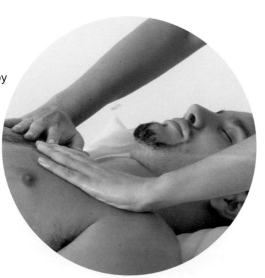

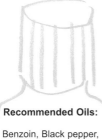

Recommended Oils:

Benzoin, Black pepper, Cajeput, Cedarwood, Cypress, Eucalyptus, Frankincense, Ginger, Lavender, Lemon, Marjoram, Myrrh, Peppermint, Rosemary, Pine, Tea tree.

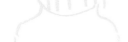

hay fever

A seasonal allergic response manifesting symptoms such as irritated watery eyes, excessive sneezing and watery nasal discharge.

Suggested aroma massage blend (to 10 ml carrier oil):

Chamomile	1 drop
Lavender	1 drop
Myrrh	1 drop

Further suggestions: avoid junk food and drink eight glasses of water daily. Learn relaxation techniques to cope with stress and eat local honey.

Recommended Oils:

Chamomile, Geranium, Lavender, Melissa, Myrrh, Immortelle, Patchouli, Yarrow.

sinusitis

Inflammation of the mucous membrane lining of the sinus cavities resulting in headaches, stuffed-up nose, mild fever and sometimes toothache and jaw pain.

Suggested aroma massage blend (to 10 ml carrier oil):

Eucalyptus	1 drop
Pine	1 drop
Tea tree	1 drop

Further suggestions: seek the advice of a practitioner trained in allergy testing; a cranial osteopath is highly recommended. Aromatherapy inhalations are excellent.

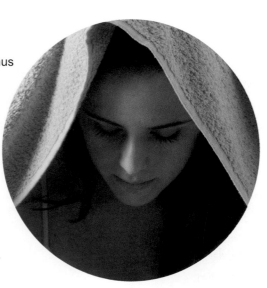

Recommended Oils:

Cajeput, Chamomile, Eucalyptus, Hyssop, Lavender, Lemon, Pine, Rosemary, Tea tree, Thyme.

throat problems

A sore throat may be due to a viral infection or overuse of the voice.

Suggested aroma massage blend (to 10 ml carrier oil):

Geranium	1 drop
Lemon	1 drop
Myrrh	1 drop

Further suggestions: gargles are a must (see page 28), rest the voice and drink lemon and honey and sage tea. Garlic capsules, zinc lozenges and the herb echinacea will all aid recovery.

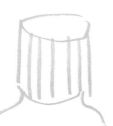

Recommended Oils:

Bergamot, Cajeput, Eucalyptus, Geranium, Ginger, Lavender, Lemon, Myrrh, Peppermint, Pine, Sage, Sandalwood, Tea tree, Thyme.

aromatherapy for the skin

acne

Acne is caused by overactivity of the sebaceous (oil-secreting) glands of the skin. The excessive sebum causes blackheads and spots, and severe acne can lead to scarring.

Suggested aroma massage blend (to 10 ml carrier oil):

Bergamot   1 drop

Carrot seed   1 drop

Chamomile   1 drop

Further suggestions: eat a well-balanced diet with plenty of fruit and vegetables. Drink eight glasses of water daily and avoid stress. Steam the face once a week, use essential oils as part of your skin care routine and dab one drop of tea tree or lavender very carefully onto spots.

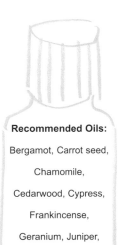

Recommended Oils:

Bergamot, Carrot seed,

Chamomile,

Cedarwood, Cypress,

Frankincense,

Geranium, Juniper,

Lemon, Lemongrass,

Patchouli, Tea tree.

ageing/mature skin

Mature skin needs moisture to ward off wrinkles and preserve its elasticity.

Suggested aroma massage blend (to 10 ml carrier oil):

Frankincense   1 drop

Neroli   1 drop

Rose   1 drop

Use petitgrain for neroli or geranium or palmarosa for rose if they are too expensive.

Recommended carrier oils: avocado pear, jojoba, or wheatgerm may be blended with apricot or peach kernel.

Further suggestions: daily facial aroma massage is essential and you should stay out of the sun. Smoking and alcohol should be avoided. Drink at least eight glasses of water daily and eat plenty of fruit, vegetables and whole grains.

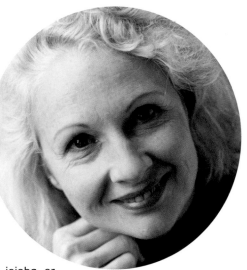

Recommended Oils:

Carrot seed,

Chamomile, Clary sage,

Frankincense,

Geranium, Jasmine,

Lavender, Neroli,

Patchouli, Rose,

Sandalwood.

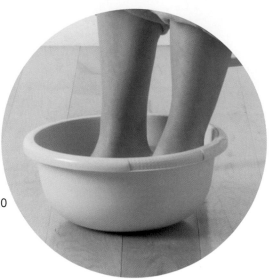

athlete's foot (tinea pedis)

A fungal condition that thrives in
between toes, causing soreness
and itching.

Suggested aroma massage blend (to 10
ml carrier oil):

Lavender	1 drop
Myrrh	1 drop
Tea tree	1 drop

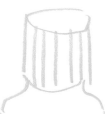

Recommended Oils:

Lavender,
Lemongrass, Myrrh,
Patchouli, Peppermint,
Tea tree.

Further suggestions: keep the feet scrupulously clean and dry, and only wear
cotton socks (no synthetic fibres). You may put neat tea tree or lavender on the
affected area. Daily aromatherapy footbaths should be taken prior to applying
the oil.

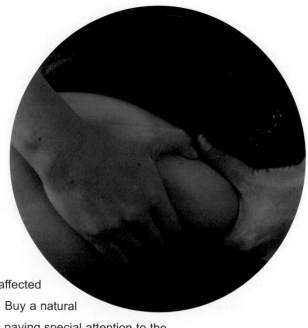

cellulite

Cellulite or 'orange peel' skin is found on the hips,
thighs and buttocks and as it affects women,
appears to be hormone-related.

Suggested aroma massage blend (to 10 ml
carrier oil):

Cypress	1 drop
Fennel	1 drop
Juniper	1 drop

Recommended Oils:

Black pepper,
Cypress, Fennel,
Ginger, Grapefruit,
Juniper, Lemon,
Lemongrass,
Rosemary, Sage.

Further suggestions: daily aroma massage of the affected
areas needs to be supported by dry skin brushing. Buy a natural
hair bristle brush and brush in upward movements paying special attention to the
cellulite. Exercise regularly and eat a diet full of fruit and vegetables and drink
eight glasses of water daily. Drink fennel tea.

cold sores (herpes simplex)

Painful sores on or near the mouth that are the result of lowered immunity, stress or excessive sunlight.

Suggested aroma massage blend (to 10 ml carrier oil):

Bergamot	1 drop
Myrrh	1 drop
Tea tree	1 drop

Further suggestions: eat a well balanced diet and take 1 gm vitamin C daily and 1000 mg lysine. You can dab neat lavender, tea tree or myrrh on the blisters. Use a gargle daily (see page 28) as a preventative measure.

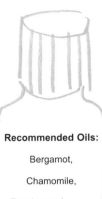

Recommended Oils:

Bergamot,

Chamomile,

Eucalyptus, Lemon,

Melissa, Myrrh,

Peppermint,

Rosemary, Tea tree.

dry skin

Dry skin is lacking in moisture and is more prone to wrinkles.

Suggested aroma massage blend (to 10 ml carrier oil):

Rose	1 drop
Neroli	1 drop
Sandalwood	1 drop

Use petitgrain for neroli or geranium or palmarosa for rose if they are too expensive. Recommended carrier oils: sweet almond, avocado pear, calendula, evening primrose, jojoba, apricot kernel, peach kernel, wheatgerm.

Further suggestions: daily aroma massage of the face is vital to 'feed' the skin. Avoid extreme heat such as hot baths and jacuzzis, as well as sunlight. Eat plenty of fruit, vegetables and oily fish, and drink at least eight glasses of water every day.

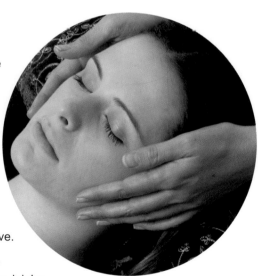

Recommended Oils:

Carrot seed,

Chamomile,

Frankincense,

Geranium, Jasmine,

Lavender, Neroli,

Rose, Sandalwood.

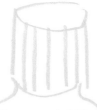

eczema

An itchy, inflammation of the skin that may be caused by allergies and diet. It most commonly affects hands, wrists and creases of the elbows or knees. There is often a family history.

Suggested aroma massage blend (to 10 ml carrier oil):

Chamomile	1 drop
Geranium	1 drop
Lavender	1 drop

Further suggestions: try to identify and avoid the allergens which can be food, cosmetics, coarse clothing or chemicals. The essential oils may also be applied in cold compresses (see page 26) to ease the intense itching and inflammation. Baking soda baths may also help – add one cup of baking soda to a tepid bath.

Recommended Oils:

Bergamot,
Cedarwood,
Chamomile,
Geranium, Juniper,
Lavender,
Frankincense, Myrrh,
Patchouli, Rose ,
Sandalwood.

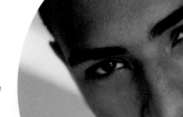

normal skin

Normal skin is smooth, fine pored, soft, supple and blemish-free.

Suggested aroma massage blend (to 10 ml carrier oil):

Chamomile	1 drop
Geranium	1 drop
Lavender	1 drop

Recommended carrier oils: sweet almond, apricot kernel, peach kernel, jojoba

Further suggestions: eat a healthy diet, exercise regularly and drink eight glasses of water daily.

Recommended Oils:

Chamomile,
Geranium, Lavender,
Neroli, Rose,
Rosewood.

oily skin

Skin that produces too much sebum due to overactive sebaceous glands is classified as oily. Pores are large and therefore prone to spots and blackheads.

Suggested aroma massage blend (to 10 ml carrier oil):

Bergamot	1 drop
Cypress	1 drop
Geranium	1 drop

Recommended carrier oils: sweet almond, apricot kernel, peach kernel, evening primrose, jojoba.

Further suggestions: avoid sugar and fatty foods, tea, coffee and tobacco. Eat plenty of fibre, fruit and vegetables and drink at least eight glasses of water daily.

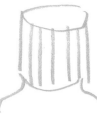

Recommended Oils:

Bergamot, Cedarwood, Cypress, Frankincense, Geranium, Juniper, Lavender, Lemon, Ylang ylang.

psoriasis

Characterised by red patches covered by scaly skin, and occurring mostly on the elbows, knees, palms of the hands, soles of the feet and the scalp. There is often a family history.

Suggested aroma massage blend (to 10 ml carrier oil):

Bergamot	1 drop
Lavender	1 drop
Yarrow or Chamomile	1 drop

Further suggestions: avoid stress which aggravates the condition. Eat a well-balanced diet incorporating oily fish. Evening primrose oil may help, as will moderate exposure to the sea and sun.

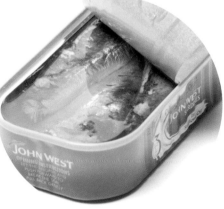

Recommended Oils:

Bergamot, Cajeput, Chamomile, Lavender, Niaouli, Yarrow.

warts and verrucae

Small abnormal growths caused by the papillomavirus affecting mostly children and young adults. Apply one of any of the recommended oils neat to the affected area. Do this two to three times daily until it disappears.

Further suggestions: eat a healthy, balanced diet, as poor nutrition can provoke an attack.

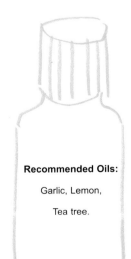

Recommended Oils:

Garlic, Lemon, Tea tree.

aromatherapy for urinary disorders

cystitis

Inflammation of the bladder characterised by painful, burning sensations when urinating, a frequent desire to urinate and possibly a low grade fever. It is usually caused by bacterial infection.

Suggested aroma massage blend (to 10 ml carrier oil):

Bergamot	1 drop
Juniper	1 drop
Lavender	1 drop

Further suggestions: regular sitz baths with any of the recommended oils (see page 25). Drink copious amounts of water and cranberry juice.

Recommended Oils:

Bergamot, Chamomile, Cajeput, Eucalyptus, Frankincense, Juniper, Lavender, Sandalwood, Tea tree.

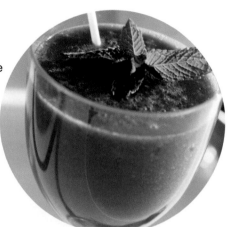

fluid retention (oedema)

Mild oedema (fluid retention) around the ankles is usually a fairly harmless condition. However, oedema should always be checked put by a doctor as it can be indicative of heart and kidney problems.

Suggested aroma massage blend (to 10 ml carrier oil):

Cypress	1 drop
Fennel	1 drop
Juniper	1 drop

Further suggestions: drink plenty of water to help flush out the kidneys. Avoid tea, coffee, alcohol and caffeine, and eat a healthy, well-balanced diet.

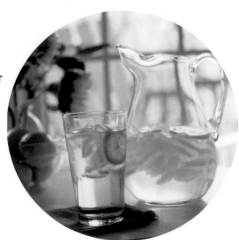

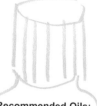

Recommended Oils:

Chamomile, Cypress, Fennel, Geranium, Juniper, Lavender, Lemon, Lemongrass, Rosemary, Sandalwood, Thyme.

useful addresses

aromatherapy suppliers

Denise Brown Essential Oils

MWB Business Exchange,

Hinton Road,

Bournemouth BH1 2EF

Tel: +44 (0)1202 708887

Fax: +44 (0)1202 708720

www.denisebrown.co.uk

A wide selection of high-quality, pure unadulterated essential oils, base oils, creams and lotions, relaxation music, wall charts, etc. is available from Denise Brown Essential Oils (International Mail Order).

aromatherapy training

Beaumont College of Natural Medicine

MWB Business Exchange,

Hinton Road,

Bournemouth,

BH1 2EF

Tel: +44 (0)1202 708887

Fax: +44 (0)1202 708720

www.beaumontcollege.co.uk

Information on training courses under the direction of Denise Brown Aromatherapy On-Line Correspondence Course www.beaumontcollege.co.uk/ correspond.html Interactive internet aromatherapy course for use on friends and family.

overseas

American Alliance of Aromatherapy

P.O. Box 750428 Petaluma,

CA 94975-0428

USA

National Association of Holistic

Aromatherapy,

P.O. Box 17622

Boulder,

CO 80308

USA

American Botanical Council

P.O. Box 201660,

Austin,

TX 78720-1660

USA

index

a

almond oil 20, 37, 121, 122, 123
angelica 10
apricot kernel 37, 119, 121, 122, 123
aroma massage 64–97, 100-124
    see also massage
aromatherapy 7
avocado oil 37, 119, 121

b

basil oil 44, 114
baths, aromatic 18–19
    footbaths 23, 120
    hand baths 23, 24
    hip 25
    sitz 25, 115, 116, 124
benzoin 24
bergamot 20, 25, 44 103, 107, 110,
116, 119, 120, 123, 124
black pepper 16, 20, 45, 100, 103, 111,
112
borage seed oil 42

c

cajeput 45, 112, 117
calendula oil 38, 121
candles 33
carrier oil 18, 22, 24, 34, 35, 36–42,
119
carrot oil 42
carrot seed 20, 119
castor oil 42
cedarwood atlas 46
chamomile 16, 20, 23, 24, 28, 46, 100,
104, 105, 106, 108, 110, 113, 118, 119,
122, 123
cider vinegar 28
circulatory disorders 47, 49, 50, 52,
53, 54, 55, 56, 58, 59, 64, 100–102

clary sage 47, 101, 115, 116
coconut oil 42
compresses 26, 27, 110, 111, 112, 113,
115, 122
cypress 25, 47, 102, 113, 114, 115, 116,
117, 120, 123, 124

d

digestive disorders 7, 44, 45, 48, 50,
52, 53, 54, 55, 56, 57, 58, 59, 60, 61, 64
103–106

e

essential oils 8–15
    absorption 16
    directory 43–61
    expression 12
    purity 13, 34
    solvent extraction 12
    steam distillation 12
    storage 14–15
eucalyptus 10, 11, 15, 48, 118
evening primrose oil 39, 121, 123

f

fennel 48, 103, 105, 106, 115, 120, 124
frankincense 20, 24, 49 101, 107, 112,
114, 117, 119
friction 75

g

gargle 28, 117, 118
garlic 16, 101, 123
geranium 24, 25, 49, 101, 102, 106,
107, 110, 114, 118, 122, 123
ginger 11, 24, 31, 50, 101, 103, 104,

106, 111, 113
grapefruit 50
grapeseed oil 39

h

haemmorroids 25, 53
hazelnut oil 42
headache 7
honey 28, 118

i

inhalations 30–31, 117, 118

j

jasmine 51, 107, 114
jojoba oil 40, 119, 121, 122, 123
juniper 24, 51, 111, 115, 120, 124

l

lavender 20, 23, 25, 52, 103, 105, 108,
109, 111, 116, 117, 118, 120, 122, 123,
124
lemon 10, 20, 28, 53, 100, 102, 103,
104, 105, 106, 112, 115, 117, 118, 123
lemongrass 54, 113
lime 109

m

macadamia oil 42
mandarin 54
marjoram 24, 55 103, 106, 109, 111,
115
massage 34 , 64–97
    abdomen 93–94
    arm 91–92

credits & acknowledgements

The author and publishers would like
to thank Alexis Henderson for
appearing as a model in this book.

picture credits

Getty Images: 7, 12, 16b, 17, 29, 100,
101m, 102t, 103, 104, 105, 106m,
108b, 109t, 112, 113b, 114, 116, 117t,
122, 124.
(b=bottom, m=middle and t=top)

Photograph p 20 by Paul Forrester

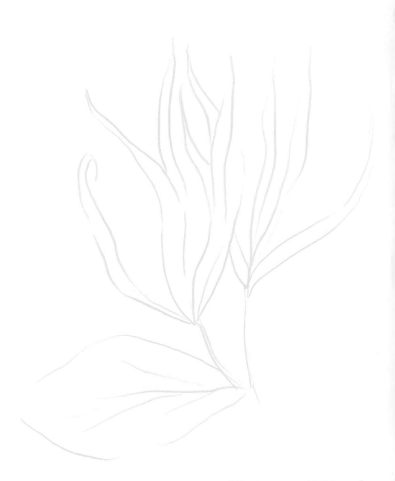